"Chaoul is a modern yogi, a man who possesses all of the technical training and cultural gifts necessary to transmit a practice that was once a hidden treasure of Bon Tibetan yoga, but is now open to any and all."

— Jeffrey J. Kripal, author of *Secret Body*

"Alejandro Chaoul has given us the gift of this powerful practice in practical easy steps. This has been a generous and lifelong devotion to bring these to the West and in particular to patients who could most benefit. This is a beautifully written and transformative book."

— Elissa Epel, Ph.D., professor, University of California, San Francisco; president elect, Academy of Behavioral Medicine Research; and best-selling co-author of *The Telomere Effect*

"*Tibetan Yoga for Health & Well-Being* is both ancient wisdom and an evidence-based clinical approach of value to anyone, whether you are living with illness or simply want to improve your sense of well-being. Alejandro Chaoul's extensive experience and passion come through in this practical guide to finding one's 'inner home' and living with openheartedness and vitality."

— Susan Bauer-Wu, Ph.D., president of the Mind & Life Institute and author of *Leaves Falling Gently*

"A wonderful combination of personal reflections, philosophy, science, and practical application. In *Tibetan Yoga for Health & Well-Being*, Alejandro Chaoul provides a narrative with specific practices to apply and help transform our daily lives."

— Lorenzo Cohen, Ph.D., professor and director, Integrative Medicine Program, the University of Texas MD Anderson Cancer Center

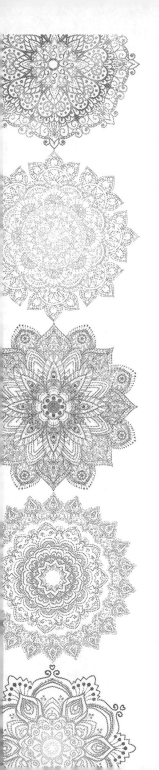

Tibetan Yoga

for Health &

Well-Being

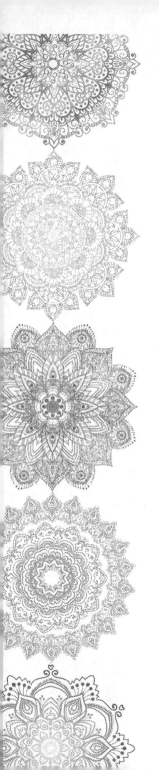

Tibetan Yoga
for Health &
Well-Being

The Science and Practice of Healing Your Body, Energy, and Mind

ALEJANDRO CHAOUL, Ph.D.

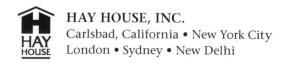

HAY HOUSE, INC.
Carlsbad, California • New York City
London • Sydney • New Delhi

Published in the United States by: Hay House, Inc.: www.hayhouse.com®
Published in Australia by: Hay House Australia Pty. Ltd.: www.hayhouse.com.au
Published in the United Kingdom by: Hay House UK, Ltd.: www.hayhouse.co.uk
Published in India by: Hay House Publishers India: www.hayhouse.co.in

Cover design: Howie Severson • *Interior design:* Bryn Starr Best

Interior photos/illustrations:
Calligraphies by Tenzin Wangyal Rinpoche
His Holiness Lungtok Tenpai Nyima, photo by Angel Alcalá
Illustrations of chakras and channels by Lhari-la Kalsang Nyima
Tibetan yoga poses in motion by Andreas Zihler, Zurich
Video of all Tibetan magical movements by Volker Graf, Vision is Mind Productions
Tibetan yoga still photos and hand details by Tom Maroshegyi

Cataloging-in-Publication Data is on file with the Library of Congress

Tradepaper ISBN: 978-1-4019-5434-5
E-book ISBN: 978-1-4019-5435-2

1st edition, July 2018

Printed in the United States of America

I dedicate this book to my teacher His Holiness
Lungtok Tenpai Nyima, the 33rd Menri Trizin, who passed away recently.

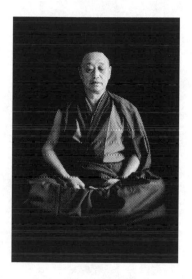

From him I first learned the Tibetan Yoga of the Instructions of the A
at his enchanting Menri Monastery in Dolanji, India, and as I write this,
I am here again for his cremation ceremony.
In the 20-plus years I studied with him, I was very fortunate to receive many
teachings, as well as my dharma name, Sherab Ozer (Wisdom Rays of Light).

Contents

Foreword

Alejandro Chaoul has been my student for more than 25 years. Over the years I have known him, he has fully engaged in Bon study and practice both academically and experientially and has played an important role in establishing some of the activities of Ligmincha International through teaching, creating support materials for practice and study, directing the research initiatives and conferences, and otherwise offering his dedicated assistance. In addition, he was in the first group of The 3 Doors trainees and is now a Senior Teacher.

From almost the beginning, he expressed interest in our *Tsa lung* and *Trul khor* Tibetan yogas, furthering his training at Triten Norbutse Monastery in Nepal and Menri Monastery in India, under the supervision of my beloved teachers Yongdzin Tenzin Namdak and His Holiness Lungtok Tenpai Nyima, respectively.

Since 1994, I have worked closely with Alejandro in the Tibetan Yoga texts and practice, supporting his teaching and trainings in the United States, Latin America, and Europe. Furthermore, with our shared interest in the healing aspect of these yogas, I was happy to support him in bringing these ancient practices into hospitals and other health-care environments, in both research and the clinic.

In *Tibetan Yoga for Health & Well-Being,* Alejandro Chaoul brings an accessible presentation of the *A-tri Trul khor,* or Tibetan Yoga of *Instructions of the A,* that we condensed together and have been teaching at Ligmincha International since 2007.

This Ligmincha 16 *A-tri Trul khor* has been met with much enthusiasm by Western students in the U.S. and internationally, and this book will be a great resource for those interested in learning about Tibetan yoga as well as for *Trul khor* practitioners around the world.

As the last chapter makes clear, this book is a resource for the modern yogi, offering different ways of connecting to one's open-heartedness for the benefit of all beings, whether you have five minutes or an hour. May these principles and practices be of benefit to many in the West as they have been for centuries in the Himalayas.

— Geshe Tenzin Wangyal Rinpoche

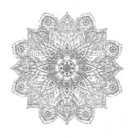

Preface

Tibetan yogis, monks, and nuns are human like you and me; they have feelings, emotions, and obstacles in their lives, like all of us. That is why the practices they have created to remove the obstacles from their body, energy, and mind are suitable for us, too. More important is that these meditative practices have enabled them to connect more deeply to themselves, and to others. And they can do this for you as well.

These ancient tools remained secret recipes for centuries, and only in the last couple of decades have they become more known in the West, been researched scientifically, and been put into practice by thousands of people. These Tibetan yogas are called *Trul khor*, which means "magical movements."

Since at least the 10th century, ancient Tibetan meditation and yogic practices have been utilized for healing the body, energy, and mind. In the 20th century, teachers such as His Holiness Lungtok Tenpai Nyima and Yongdzin Tenzin Namdak Rinpoche preserved these teachings by risking their lives to bring them to safety in India and training many *geshes* (the equivalent of having a Ph.D./Th.D., a doctorate in philosophy or theology, in Bon and Buddhist Studies) and yogis at Menri Monastery, as well as at Triten Norbutse Monastery in Nepal. Among these geshes was Tenzin Wangyal Rinpoche, with whom I had the great fortune and blessing to train, as well as his teachers (mentioned above) and other wonderful teachers like Lopon Trinley Nyima and Khenpo Tenpa Yungdrung. Since 1999, we have been utilizing these yogic practices at the University of Texas MD Anderson Cancer Center in Houston and at other hospitals under the supervision of Tenzin Wangyal Rinpoche.

The material for this book stems from over a decade of work, including my Ph.D. dissertation on Tibetan yoga and its applications in contemporary health care settings.[1] I first learned of Tibetan yogic practices in the early 1990s, and since then I have been practicing and continuing to learn. With the authorization of Tenzin Wangyal Rinpoche, I have taught these practices for over 20 years to students that included cancer patients, their families, and their caregivers.

My goal is to help you learn how to remove obstacles in your everyday life by applying powerful ancient Tibetan yogic methods of body, energy, and mind. The five principal breaths of Tibetan medicine and yoga can become the five main principles in your everyday life, bringing you health and well-being.

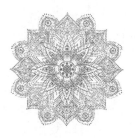

Introduction

The year 2000 was very special for many reasons. In fact, it was a pregnant year, both metaphorically and literally. Tenzin Wangyal Rinpoche organized a retreat honoring his teacher, Yongdzin Tenzin Namdak, in Kathmandu, Nepal. Participants had the wonderful opportunity to enter this millennium with them, to visit Yongdzin Rinpoche's monastery, Triten Norbutse, and meet the monks, and to see many places in Kathmandu and its surroundings.

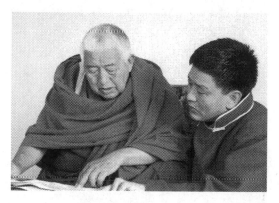

Yongdzin Tenzin Wangyal and Tenzin Wangyal Rinpoche
at Triten Norbutse in 2000. Photo by author.

I was so happy that my wife, Erika, joined me at the retreat, and that we brought along our 16-month-old son, Matías Namdak. Erika's sister, Katy, also joined us. It was a very meaningful and magical trip, one that reawakened much of my spiritual journey. Among the magical moments was the one when we realized that Erika was pregnant. Nine months later, on September 1, Karina Dawa was born.

After that retreat, my family went back to the United States while I stayed in Triten Norbutse for another month to continue learning Tibetan yoga and deepening my practice by joining the *drubdra*, or meditation group. I felt very blessed to be able to join this small group of Tibetan monks, and to have the marvelous opportunity to learn more from Yongdzin Rinpoche. This was the same monastery where almost a decade before I had first learned the Tibetan yogas, or magical movements, from the Bon tradition.

After returning to the United States, the magazine *Yoga Journal* interviewed me and published an article on Tibetan yoga by Elaine Lipson. Called "Into the Mystic," it brought attention to the fact that in the West, Tibetan yoga was very little known and largely unavailable, yet there was growing curiosity about and interest in it. In 2007, Lipson wrote a follow-up article called "Unraveling the Mystery of Tibetan Yoga Practices" that pointed out how very few centers and teachers in the West were openly teaching these Tibetan yogas. She highlighted the Dzogchen Community, led by Namkhai Norbu Rinpoche and the Ligmincha Institute, led by Tenzin Wangyal Rinpoche, underscoring that they teach Tibetan yogas from the original, authentic texts and sources.

One of the challenges that these teachers faced was maintaining the authenticity of these practices while bringing them to a larger audience in a way that was accessible. Both Namkhai Norbu Rinpoche and Tenzin Wangyal Rinpoche understand this tension and deliver their teachings with this in mind. I have been very fortunate to be trained by both of them, and when I began to teach, I took their advice to heart. Namkhai Norbu Rinpoche emphasized the importance of the five elements, particularly in the Bon tradition. With Tenzin Wangyal Rinpoche, I learned how the five elements have correlations with the five kinds of breath-energy—as we will see in this book—and how the Tibetan yogas bring them into one's practice.

As I was writing my Ph.D. dissertation, "Magical Movements: Tibetan Yoga from the Ancient Bon Tradition and Applications in Contemporary Medicine," I went to do my fieldwork at Menri Monastery in India to learn the Tibetan Yoga of *Instructions of the A* under the tutelage of His Holiness Lungtok Tenpai Nyima. He was firm in asking me to come for the classic 100-day retreat, but Karina was a year old and Matías was three, so leaving them for over three months would have been very difficult. Erika and I decided I could go for two months, and when I called His Holiness to say that I could only come for 60 days, he responded, "When are you arriving?"

I took daily teachings with His Holiness and also with Lopon Trinley Nyima, the main teacher (*lopon*) at Menri Monastery. It was an intense and wonderful time of study and practice, without which I could not be writing this book.

Since earning my Ph.D., I have been teaching in various settings, from academia, to hospitals, to meditation centers, to yoga studios. I am also part of the Integrative Medicine Center at MD Anderson Cancer Center, where we research the benefits of these practices and then bring them into the clinic. Through Ligmincha International, I continue to train individuals in the United States, Latin America, and Europe who are interested in deepening their Tibetan yoga practice through multiyear trainings.

What Is Tibetan Yoga?

Yoga is a global phenomenon that is practiced today in a variety of places, from gyms, to yoga studios, to temples, to many Western homes. For the most part, these are mind-body practices that have their origin in India, some emphasizing body posture (*asana*), others breathing practices (*pranayama*), and still others mind or meditation practices. In the practice of these Indian-based yogas, the practitioner brings the body into a specific posture, allowing the breath to flow and the mind to settle.

In the mind-body practices that originated in China, usually called *Qigong* and *T'ai Chi*, the practitioner learns to move the body in sync with the breath-energy (*qi*) and the mind settles into that flow.

The Tibetan yogas, *Tsa lung* and *Trul khor* (magical movements of breath and channels), are distinctive mind-energy-body practices where the practitioner brings their mind and breath together and, while holding them still, moves the body in a particular way to direct that breath-energy in five distinct ways, then exhales and settles their mind in a radical sense of full awareness. The special quality of awareness arising from these mind—breath-energy—body movements is why they are called magical movements.

Written texts describing these magical movements trace back to the 10th century, but they reportedly were transmitted orally long before that.

Trul, which is usually translated as "magic" or "magical," can also take on the meaning of "machine" or "mechanics." *Khor* means "wheel," but also "circular movement" or just "movement." Therefore, *Trul khor* can be translated as "magical movement(s)" or "magical wheel," and sometimes "spinning the machinery with wheels or chakras."[1] Khenpo Tenpa Yungdrung, current abbot of Triten Norbutse Monastery in Nepal, says that *trul* in the Tibetan yoga context refers to the magic of "the unusual effects that these movements produce in the experience of the practitioner."[2]

Not Just Mind-Body, but Mind–Breath–Energy–Body

Although mainstream Western medicine has not totally recognized or embraced the connection between physical illness and energetic or mental obstacles, there are new paradigms in the emerging field of complementary and integrative medicine (CIM) that do acknowledge it and are more akin to and congruent with Asian systems. In fact, beginning in the 1930s and flourishing especially from the 1970s onward, "more than a thousand studies of meditation have been reported in English-language journals, books, and graduate theses."[3]

Over the last decade and a half I have engaged in researching the possible practical and physical applications of these Tibetan mind-body techniques in a Western medical setting.[4] In particular, I have focused on the potential benefits of Tibetan yoga as part of CIM treatments for cancer patients.

When I met Lorenzo Cohen, Ph.D., then a behavioral researcher at the University of Texas MD Anderson Cancer Center in Houston and now director of their Integrative Medicine Program, in 2000, he asked me to design a Tibetan yoga intervention for cancer patients. We formed a team and began conducting randomized, controlled clinical trials to determine the feasibility, acceptability, and initial efficacy of these practices. Our findings have been published in various journals.[5, 6, 7, 8, 9, 10, 11]

In Tibetan Buddhist and Bon teachings, one's physical body, breath, and mind are known as the three doors through which one practices and realizes enlightenment. Within the speech or energy realm, a subtle energy body emerges metaphorically and, for some, in actuality. In Tibetan, this "subtle body" is composed of channels (*tsa*) that help guide the breath-energy (*lung*—pronounced loong—called *prana* in the Indian yogas and *qi* in Chinese mind-body practices). This subtle body provides the landscape where the mind and the physical body connect with each other through the five breath-energies.

As you will learn in Chapters 1 and 2, in the Tibetan yoga practices, you become familiar with the channels first through visualization and then by using your mind to direct the breath along those channels as you familiarize yourself with each kind of breath-energy. In this way, you guide your breath-energy through your channels more evenly in terms of the rhythm of the inhalation and exhalation and seek greater balance in the amount and strength of the breath.

A well-known ancient Tibetan metaphor describes the mind riding on the breath-energy like a rider upon a horse, with the two traveling together through the pathways of the channels. So, as the breath-energy circulating through the channels becomes more balanced, the channels become increasingly flexible, allowing the breath-energy to find its own comfortably smooth rhythm. When the breath rhythm is smooth, like a wave, the mind has a smoother ride, which reduces the tendency to become agitated. With the help of movements that guide the mind and the five kinds of breath-energies into different areas of the body and energy centers, or chakras, the practice brings the possibility of healing or harmonizing body, breath-energy, and mind— which we can call the body–breath-energy–mind system. This is a goal of yogic practices, and also a model of good health that is in line with the concept of health or well-being in Tibetan medicine.

Tibetan Yoga and Tibetan Medicine: Bringing Health through Balancing the Five Elements and Our Five Breath-Energies *(Lung)*

Tibetan medical texts explain the "science of healing" *(sowa rigpa)*, or Tibetan medicine, in terms of the balancing of one's internal constitution defined by the three medical "humors"—wind, bile, and phlegm—and the five elements—earth, water, fire, air, and space. Health is not solely the concern with regard to physical illness or disease. Instead, the harmony of the body, breath-energy, and mind system is most important.

Among the three humors, the "wind" humor, *lung* in Tibetan, is described as having five distinct kinds of breath-energies, for which the important Bon text *Mother Tantra*, describes as a set of five channel-breath *(tsa lung)* yogic movements. Each movement is explained in terms of those same five breath-energies described in the Tibetan medical system and is correlated with the five elements. This is equivalent to the five *pranas* or *vayus* in the Indian medical system of ayurveda. The Tibetan Yoga of *Instructions of the A* also follows the five-*lung* or breath-energy system, its relationships to the elements, and how it can balance your body, breath-energy, and mind. In fact, **these five breath-energies are the five vital breath principles at the foundation of Tibetan yoga for health and well-being.**

After I had been facilitating a Tibetan meditation class for a year at the Place of Wellness (now called the Integrative Medicine Center) at the University of Texas MD Anderson Cancer Center, Dr. Lorenzo Cohen asked me to propose a research "intervention" based on the Tibetan mind-body practices. I wanted to make sure it addressed the whole person and was true to the Tibetan mind-body healing practices. After asking for the approval and support of my Tibetan teachers in using these practices, I joined a research team led by Dr. Cohen with the aim of investigating the possible benefits of a Tibetan mind-body intervention in people with cancer.[12]

This first Tibetan mind-body intervention centered on the five breath-energy and channel (*Tsa lung*) mind-body practices, which emphasize the five breath-energies and the five elements, and *Trul khor* yogic movements, which work with the whole body–breath-energy–mind continuum.

We had an opportunity to present this Tibetan yoga intervention for people with cancer in 1998 at the First International Congress on Tibetan Medicine, in Washington, D.C. It was the first time that Lorenzo Cohen and Tenzin Wangyal Rinpoche met in person. As the three of us were discussing the development of our study and how to look into the future, Lorenzo asked Rinpoche what change in participating patients he would consider most important. Without hesitation, Rinpoche said, "Openheartedness."

As you practice this yoga with awareness, breath-energy, and movements, you will notice that you will become more centered.

This centeredness can be felt in the central channel and in the chakras, particularly in the main chakra—the heart—and you, too, can experience this openheartedness.

Healing, Mystical, or Magical?

The Tibetan yoga texts state that through your practice, you balance your elements, making the whole body function like a well-oiled machine. With your body a cleansed receptacle and functioning well, the mind's awareness gains lucidity that is expressed throughout the body, energy, and mind. It is in this way that these movements are magical, says Khenpo Tenpa Yungdrung, abbot of Triten Norbutse Monastery in Kathmandu, Nepal, and of the Shenten Dargye Ling center in France. In other words, these Tibetan yogic practices can be understood as movements that manipulate the body, breath, and mind, which can lead to internal or even mystical experiences and the development of a radical awareness of one's own natural state of being by stripping away the layers of obstacles of body, energy, and mind. This is what is sometimes known as a spiritual transformation, and it may be similar to what the famous Chinese philosopher and mystic Lao-tzu expressed:

> Bodily shifts, however multiple or spectacular, are but incidental to the internal transformation experienced. It is internal transformation at the deepest level that becomes the most sought after religious experience.[13]

The Instructions of the A, in fact, means instructions for rediscovering or reconnecting to your natural or primordial state of mind, which is calm, open, and luminous.

In 2007, Tenzin Wangyal Rinpoche asked me to help condense the Tibetan Yoga of *Instructions of the A* with two geshes, Tenzin Yangton and Tenzin Yeshe, during the Ligmincha Institute's Annual Summer Retreat in Virginia. During the three-week retreat, we met daily to condense the 40 movements of the original text into what is in this book. Sometimes I call them the Ligmincha *A-tri Trul khor*, or simply the Ligmincha 16, since there are 16 movements—one foundational and 15 principal. The principal movements are subdivided into the 5 breath-energies, with 3 movements for each of the 5, for a total of 15.

As you practice the magical movements of Tibetan yoga, you can reproduce or alter your experiences by guiding your breath-energy, enabling you to connect with your natural state of mind, or what I like to call your "inner home," represented by the crystal-clear *A*. In Tibetan, the syllable A, represents one's calm, open, and luminous state of mind. And many times it is white or crystal clear, illustrating that open and luminous aspect. Using this Tibetan yoga, you can generate specific experiences and be an active participant in your own healing and your life.

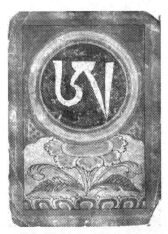

Ancient Tibetan ritual card (tsakli)
representing the crystal-clear A

CHAPTER 1

The Ligmincha Yoga of
Instructions of the A

Tibetan Yoga for Everyone
and Everyday Life

THE LIGMINCHA YOGA OF *INSTRUCTIONS OF THE A* practice consists of stating your purpose or intention, using proper body posture and breathings, understanding your subtle body with inner channels and guiding your breath through them, and, finally, incorporating the magical movements. I will present it in five steps, three (intention, posture and breathings, and subtle body) in this chapter, and then the fourth and fifth, the magical movements and sharing the benefits of your practice, in Chapter 2.

STEP 1: Stating Your Purpose or Intention

The *Instructions of the A* yoga text starts with a beautiful Tibetan homage that describes the intention we cultivate when we practice this yoga:

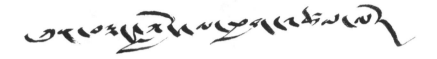

Kun zang long la chag tsal lo

This *praises being in the expanse of one's natural state of mind,* which is reached by clearing the external and internal obstacles with this Tibetan yoga practice. The main purpose of this practice is to achieve that fully aware and focused *A state of mind.*

It is important to first calm one's "monkey mind," the aspect of the mind that goes from thought to thought and emotion to emotion like a monkey from one branch to the next in search of happiness.

Traditionally, the practices called *zhiné,* or calm abiding, focus your attention on an object—external or internal—which allows your mind to relax, concentrate, and connect to yourself more deeply.

Over 40 years ago, Herbert Benson, M.D., at Harvard Medical School scientifically proved that a simple breathing meditation can elicit what he called the *relaxation response.*[1] During the relaxation response, a series of changes occur that increase the activity of your parasympathetic nervous system to balance the "fight or flight" response that heightens the activity of your sympathetic nervous system and provokes a cascade of brain chemicals that our body perceives as stress. In other words, the relaxation response is a decrease in physiological stress that helps you achieve a state of calm. Therefore, learning how to breath properly is very important for practicing this yoga, and for your everyday life.

When I started teaching meditation at the MD Anderson Cancer Center almost 20 years ago, in consultation with my teachers and the hospital, I designed a simple meditation practice that I called Connecting with Your Heart. It helps you relax your monkey mind, notice and adjust your body posture, and focus on your breathing, thereby enhancing your connection to your mind-heart, your inner home.

STEP 2: Using Proper Body Posture and Breathings

Your body posture is key in sustaining your mind's attention on your breath. As you prepare to meditate, focusing on your body posture can bring a sense of stillness that aids in attaining the stillness and focus of your mind; your breath becomes the link between your body and mind.

The preferred posture for this practice is the classic meditation posture that has five points.

The Five-Point Posture

On a cushion or mat:

- Sit cross-legged, which helps to contain your warmth and energy within your body and helps you keep your back straight.

- Keep your back straight, which aids the flow of energy and keeps the channels straight.

- Make your chest open, like an eagle soaring in the sky, to give yourself a sense of openness and lightness so you are not too tense.

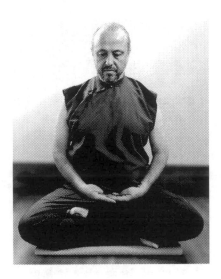

- Hold your hands in the equipoise position (palms up, left palm resting on right, thumbs at the bases of the corresponding ring fingers, resting on your lap), which supports an inner sense of equanimity.

- Tuck your jaw slightly down and in to lengthen the back of your neck and lessen the wandering of your thoughts.

If you are unable to sit on a cushion on the floor, you may sit in a chair with your feet flat on the floor. Keep your back straight and sit toward the edge of the chair. The rest of the pose is the same, as set out above.

Keep your eyes closed or, if you prefer to keep them open, gaze downward peacefully without looking around.

Conscious Breathing

A simple way to start your breathing, with your mind guiding your breath, is to:

1. **Inhale/breathe in**—Welcome all positive and nurturing qualities.

2. **Exhale/breathe out**—Let go of negative and obstructive qualities.

3. **Relax**—Find an inner space where you feel more connected to yourself.

Guided Practice: Connecting with Your Heart

Now that you have set the intention of your practice of staying connected with your mind-heart for the benefit of all beings by clearing external and internal obstacles, and that you know the correct posture and have performed a simple breathing exercise, here is a guided practice that incorporates these aspects and concludes with sharing the benefits of your practice with all beings.

Connecting with Your Heart guided practice (approx. 10 to 12 minutes)

Read the text below to support your practice. If you would like an audio recording of it, see Resources (page 87), where you'll find a link to the free audio files that I have used with positive results in the clinic at MD Anderson and in my research.

Welcome,

Take a moment to sit comfortably on your cushion or chair.

Take a deep and comfortable breath.

Feel comfortable in your body posture, exhaling any stress.

Keep your body straight but also relaxed, and as you breathe in and out, connect to the stillness that your body provides.

Allow your shoulders to relax, but keep your back straight.

Relax your forehead, jaw, and face with a gentle smile as you bring your tongue up to your upper palate. Breathe comfortably, if possible through your nose.

Relax your eyes, closing them if that's comfortable. If you prefer them open, look at the tip of your nose and down into the floor.

Maintaining your mind's attention on your breath, keep inhaling and exhaling through your nose, slowly bringing your breath lower into your abdomen, letting it inflate like a balloon with the inhalation, and contract comfortably with the exhalation. If your mind gets distracted, gently bring it back to your breath.

Our mind can be like a monkey jumping from branch to branch as it follows thoughts or is distracted by sounds, so without judgment, bring your awareness back to your breath, breathing into your abdomen and back to your nose. As we use our breath to connect, our breath becomes our anchor.

Take a few soft, gentle breaths, keeping your mind's attention on your breath.

You can visualize your breath as light. As you breathe in, feel that your breath brings nurturing qualities with that light. These nurturing qualities could be physical, emotional, mental, or spiritual, and allow yourself to receive that nourishment. As you exhale, breathe out any obstacles or discomforts—any tensions, fear, negativity, pain—anything that no longer serves you. Let it go in that exhalation. And as you feel more comfortable, more settled at home, enjoy that stillness.

Now, listen to the silence instead of letting your mind follow sounds or thoughts. As you connect to your inner silence, you may feel a sense of inner peace.

Let your breath be an invitation to stay in the present moment and rest in that silence, allowing any obstacle to pass by like a bird flying in the sky, leaving no trace. In that inner sacred space and the support of the silence, your awareness dawns like the sun illuminating that space, and with that light, feel its warmth. Breathe and connect more deeply to that warmth.

This warmth can be your loving kindness, your compassion, your inner joy.

Connect deeply from your heart as you keep on breathing.

And as you feel more connected to yourself, open your heart and allow this feeling to connect you to others. Share all the wonderful qualities you now feel. It is like pouring nectar into the ocean, so that everyone, including you, can drink, and be nourished from those qualities.

Feel the openness of your inner space, your awareness as light, and your warmth as your loving kindness, compassion, and inner joy, sharing it with others and yourself.

Rest in that state for a few moments.

And as you maintain that sense of connection, without needing to open your eyes yet, you can slowly start to relax your body. Stretch your legs, your arms, and relax your body. Relax all the muscles of your face, your jaw; relax your eyes . . . and take your time to slowly open your eyes. Integrate with the external world, slowly breathing, without losing touch of your inner home, and remember that you can maintain this state of mind in your everyday life.

Every breath is an opportunity to connect in this way. Stay connected.

Have a wonderful day!

Nine Breathings of Purification

Breath is the most palpable aspect of our energy, so working more with our breath helps us to be more in tune with the mind-energy-body connection.

In addition to the way we use breath in Connecting with Your Heart, a more traditional Tibetan and elaborate breathing practice that you can use is called the **Nine Breathings of Purification**. At MD Anderson, we use it in our Power of Breath class, as well as in the Tibetan yoga research protocols.

Nine Breathings of Purification consists of three kinds of breaths. You repeat each kind three times using alternate-nostril breathing, and then breathe through both nostrils to clear the three poisons or afflictions that do not allow us to be in our meditative state—anger, attachment, and confusion. Once we clear these, we can be more open in our connection to our inner home and feel more balanced. From the Tibetan medicine perspective, this inner balance brings health of body, energy, and mind.

Breath is a wonderful tool for clearing your external and internal obstacles. Like the wind removing the clouds and letting us see the sky that was already there, these breathings can remove anger, attachment, and confusion, which the Tibetan medical and yogic traditions hold are the chief afflictions that prevent you from being healthy and realizing your natural state of mind.

Think about how anger can hijack you. When you are angry, you almost become anger itself, and you say, "I am angry." You then see all the things around you through the lens of anger, limiting your perspective and your ability to be open to yourself and to others. Similarly, when you are attached to something or the way in which something has turned out, you limit yourself by not being able to "unstick" yourself from that situation or allow yourself to be in a more open state of mind. Finally, confusion is a muddy or cloudy state of mind that prevents you from clearly seeing what is really going on, and thus it limits your perspective with a lack of clarity.

Therefore, once you have calmed and focused your mind using the Connecting with Your Heart meditation, you will be able to fully engage in the Nine Breathings of Purification and connect to your breath for balance, clearing your obstacles and helping you gear up for the magical movements.

First set of three breaths: **Purifying Anger**

- Place your right thumb at the base of your ring finger.

- Close your right nostril with your right hand's ring finger.

- Breathe in through your left nostril and feel your breath energizing the left side of your body.

- Release your right nostril, and, reaching across your face, cover your left nostril with your right hand's ring finger.

- Exhale completely through your right nostril to dissolve obstacles related to anger.

- Repeat for a total of three rounds, inhaling through your left nostril and exhaling through your right nostril.

- Notice how you feel—maybe a little more open—on the right side of your body.

Second set of three breaths: **Purifying Attachment**

- Place your left thumb at the base of your ring finger.
- Close your left nostril with your left hand's ring finger.
- Breathe in through your right nostril and feel the breath energizing the right side of your body.
- Release your left nostril and, reaching across your face, cover your right nostril with your left hand's ring finger.
- Exhale completely through your left nostril to dissolve obstacles related to attachment.
- Repeat for a total of three rounds, inhaling through the right nostril and exhaling through the left nostril.
- Notice how you feel—maybe a little more open—on the left side of your body.

Third set of three breaths: **Purifying Confusion or Self-Doubt**

- Place your hands on your lap in the equipoise position, left over right, palms up, and thumbs at the bases of the ring fingers.
- Breathe in through both nostrils and feel the breath energizing your whole body.
- Exhale completely through both nostrils, dissolving obstacles related to confusion or self-doubt.

- Repeat for a total of three rounds, inhaling and exhaling through both nostrils.

- Notice how you feel—maybe a little more open—in your whole body.

After practicing the Nine Breathings of Purification and clearing obstacles within yourself, rest in a meditative state, staying relaxed and alert in your inner home. Remain comfortable within this experience for a few minutes, and then, to conclude, come back to your heart center and actualize your intention by sharing the benefits of your practice with others and with yourself.

STEP 3: Subtle-Body Practice: Incorporating Your Channels and Guiding Your Breath through Them

The subtle energy body, as its name suggests, is a subtler awareness of the body achieved by using the mind's attention to guide the breath-energy through it. The breath-energy becomes a crucial link between your experience of your mind and body. When you do practices like the Nine Breathings of Purification, you can amplify their potency by performing them with the support of your subtle body. There are many conceptions of the subtle body. The one that is used in this Tibetan yoga consists of three main channels and five energy centers, or chakras.

The numbers and locations of the chakras vary by tradition and even by specific practice, but in general, the most important ones are located along the central channel, right in front of and along your spinal chord. Shardza Tashi Gyaltsen Rinpoche, a famous 19th-century Bon scholar and teacher, described them as:

- Crown, the chakra of great bliss, located at the top of your head

- Throat, the chakra of enjoyment and experience

- Heart, the chakra of your true nature

- Navel, the chakra of manifestation

- Secret, the chakra that sustains bliss, located at your perineum

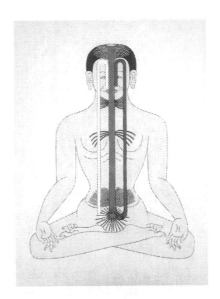

The Tibetan yoga of the *Instructions of the A* will help you engage one or more chakras at a time, clearing obstructions and eliciting the different experiences in your different chakras. These movements relate to the five kinds of breath-energies that are identified in Tibetan medicine. When the breath is brought to each of the five chakras, it expresses the energy of that chakra as one of the five breath-energies, helping you to release obstacles, feel openness, and provide nurturing at different levels.

Your channels and chakras, and the breath-energies circulating through them, make up the subtle "playground" needed for the body movements in the poses of Tibetan yoga. In each of the poses you hold your breath, often in one of your chakras, while you move your body in a way that directs that breath, which has been guided by your mind.

Now that you know a little bit more about your subtle body and your channels, let's again explore the Nine Breathings of Purification, but now with the assistance of your channels.

Nine Breathings of Purification with Channels

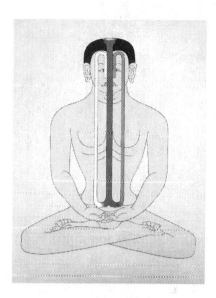

Right Channel, Central Channel, and Left Channel.

When working to clear obstacles using the breathing practices, imagine the three main channels of the body: the central channel and the two side channels, the right and the left. These channels are made of light.

- The central channel, which you can visualize as blue light, rises straight along the center of your body and in front of your spinal chord, widens slightly from your heart to its opening at the top of your head. It is described as being the diameter of a bamboo cane.

- The two side or secondary channels are somewhat smaller in diameter and join with the central channel at its base, about four finger-widths below your navel.

You can visualize them with colors if that helps
you focus on them, with the left one red and the
right one white. These side channels rise straight
up from the junction with the central channel,
running parallel at the right and left of the central
channel. However, whereas the central channel rises
through the top of your head, the side channels
curve around just under the top of your skull, pass
downward behind the eyes, and then open at the
corresponding nostrils.

- The right (white) channel represents method (*skillful means*) or qualities. This is the channel of the male energies.

- The left (red) channel represents wisdom. It is the channel of the female energies.

- *The central channel is the main pathway.* It is not a physical road or highway. Instead, it is a path, a stream of consciousness. In terms of experience, it is hard to define the central channel. There is no ordinary terminology for it. The simplest way to express it is to say it is a deep sense of settling within yourself, being completely at rest with full awareness rather than sleeping. We all know how to sleep, but resting with full awareness is something you must learn how to do.

- The chakras, which lie along the central channel, present opportunities for you to connect with certain qualities and characteristics to enhance your practice and your life. (See page 12.)

A link to video recordings of a guided practice for the Nine Breathings of Purification is in the Resources section (page 87).

Exercising the Pathways of the Secondary Channels

Sit in the five-point posture (page 4) or comfortably on a chair and visualize the central and secondary channels.

Before we engage in the Nine Breathings of Purification again, familiarize yourself with guiding your breath through your channels. To do so:

- Breathe in and out through both nostrils as you did in the third set of breathing described earlier (pages 10–11).

- Continue breathing in and out through both nostrils and guide your breath from your nostrils to your side channels, using the channels as pathways for your breath-energy. Let your mind's awareness guide your breath to carry your nurturing qualities in the inhalation and remove your obstacles in the exhalation.

- Repeat this process several times, inhaling and exhaling through both nostrils.

I have found it very useful, both for myself and when teaching, to do this simple breathing exercise to get familiar with my two side channels before beginning the Nine Breathings of Purification practice.

As you practice the Nine Breathings using your side channels, focus on releasing your main affliction and recognizing the space within and calmness of your mind after that release. Every time you inhale, visualize the air as a green light, since green is the color of the air element. During the exhalation, visualize the air as smoke to represent letting go of your afflictions. Anger or irritation are represented as blue smoke, attachment or control as pink smoke, and confusion or self-doubt as gray smoke. Note that when using the channels in the third set of breaths, you will guide your breath-energy through your central channel and crown chakra, although, of course, your normal, physical breath will be exhaled through your nostrils.

Guided Practice of the Nine Breathings of Purification, Incorporating Your Channels

PREPARATION:
Now that you are more familiar with your subtle body's channels and guiding your breath-energy through them, you are again ready to engage in the Nine Breathings of Purification. Use the three kinds of breath with the support of your channels to purify your emotions of anger, attachment, and confusion.

Sitting in the five-point posture (page 4) or in a chair, bring your mind's attention to your breath. As you breathe in and out a few times, visualize your three channels.

The first three breaths: **Purifying Anger**

- Place your right thumb at the base of your right ring finger.

- Close your right nostril with that ring finger.

- Inhale through your left nostril, feeling the pure, nourishing air coming into your body.

- Imagine the breath as green light following your left channel.

- As your breath travels through your left channel, feel how your channel expands, like a balloon being inflated.

- As your breath reaches the point of union of your channels, allow it to continue to your right side, and slowly release your right ring finger from your right nostril and close your left nostril with that same finger.

- Guide your breath as it follows your right channel up your body and out through your right nostril, visualizing it as dark blue smoke and feeling this releasing breath carrying blocks and obstacles, especially those related to anger, from your body, energy, and mind.

- Imagine these obstacles dissolving instantly into the vast surrounding space.

- Repeat two more times. In the inhalation, breathe in pure air through your left nostril and left channel, visualizing it as green light, to nourish and support your concentration. Then feel that air traverse your right channel and, in the exhalation through your right nostril, visualize it as dark blue smoke, carrying out the obstacles of anger to let them out of your system.

- Take a moment to notice how you feel on your right side and right channel—maybe a sense of being more open and possibly a little less anger or irritation.

The second three breaths: **Purifying Attachment**

- Place your left thumb at the base of your left ring finger.

- Close your left nostril with that ring finger.

- Inhale through your right nostril, feeling the pure, nourishing air coming into your body.

- Imagine the breath as green light following the path of your right channel.

- As your breath travels through your right channel, feel how your channel expands, like a balloon being inflated.

- As your breath reaches the point of union of your channels, allow it to continue to your left side, and slowly release your left ring finger from your left nostril and close your right nostril with that same finger.

- Guide your breath as it follows your left channel up your body and out through your left nostril, visualizing it as pink smoke and feeling this releasing breath carrying blocks and obstacles, especially those related to desire and attachment, from your body, energy, and mind.

- Imagine these obstacles dissolving instantly into the vast surrounding space.

- Repeat two more times. In the inhalation, breathe in pure air, visualizing it as green light, through your right nostril and your right channel, to nourish and support your concentration. Then feel it traverse the left channel and, in the exhalation through your left nostril, visualizing the air as pink smoke, breathe out the obstacles of attachment to let them out of your system.

- Take a moment to notice how you feel on your left side and left channel   maybe a sense of being more open and possibly a little less grasping, attachment or control.

The third three breaths: **Purifying Confusion or Cloudy Mind**

- Place your hands on your lap in the equipoise position, left over right, with the palms up and the thumbs at the bases of the ring fingers.

- Inhale through both nostrils, feeling the pure, nourishing air coming into your body.

- Imagine the breath as green light following your right and left side channels.

- As your breath travels through them, feel how the channels expand, like balloons being inflated.

- As your breath reaches the point of union of your channels, allow it to enter and continue up your central channel as you guide it along the pathway. Feel the subtle breath going up your central channel and leaving slightly upward through your crown chakra, visualizing it as dark gray smoke. Exhale your normal physical breath through your nostrils.

- Feel this releasing breath carrying blocks and obstacles, especially those related to confusion or unawareness, from your body, energy, and mind.

- Imagine these obstacles dissolving instantly into the vast surrounding space.

- Repeat two more times. In the inhalation, breathe in pure air through both nostrils, visualizing it as green light, to nourish and support your concentration. In the exhalation, visualizing the air as dark smoke, breathe out the obstacles slightly upward through your crown chakra and also through both nostrils.

- Take a moment to notice how you feel in your central channel and your whole body—maybe a sense of being more open, and a little less cloudy mind and more clarity instead.

Now, having deeply nurtured and purified yourself, rest in your inner home while you get ready to connect to your chakras and start the Tibetan yoga movements.

An Experiential Run through the Chakras: Preparing the Energy Landscape[2]

This practice brings your attention to each of your energy centers— chakras—so you can open to the subtle movement of the five breath-energies that circulate in your subtle body.

This will help you become familiar with having your mind carry your breath through the channels and the chakras as you familiarize yourself with each breath-energy that you will eventually incorporate into the Tibetan yoga movements.

As you breathe into each chakra, hold your breath comfortably in that chakra for a few seconds so you can feel its energy there, and then slowly release, noticing how you feel before going on to the next chakra. At the end, one simple movement will bring the pervasive breath-energy expanding throughout your channels and chakras and clearing through every pore of your body, leaving you open and ready for the Tibetan yoga movements.

Guided Practice through the Five Chakras and Pervasive Breath Exercise

1. Focus your attention on your breath filling your *throat chakra*. As you slightly hold your breath there, feel any experience that arises as you allow that breath to move upward toward your crown chakra. Feel your breath waking up and nourishing your sense organs, then reaching your *crown chakra*. Notice how you feel there and exhale slightly upward (as you did in the third kind of breathing in the Nine Breathings of Purification on pages 19–20). Take a moment to notice how you feel in your throat and crown chakras.

2. Now, slowly bring your attention and breath down to your *heart chakra*. Hold your breath slightly as you contact the life force–sustaining energy of your mind-heart. After a few seconds, exhale slowly, as if your heart chakra is a valve for releasing air, subtle air, and unwanted energy out the front and back. Notice how you feel in your heart chakra.

3. Slowly bring your attention and breath down to your *navel chakra*. Hold your breath slightly as you connect

to your fire energy of digestion and creativity, then exhale slowly, as if your navel chakra is also a valve for releasing the air, subtle air, and unwanted energy out the front and back. Notice how you feel in your navel chakra.

4. Slowly bring your attention and breath down to your *secret chakra* (inside yourself, at your perineum, within the space between your anus and genitals). Hold your breath slightly, connecting to your blissful downward and clearing moving energy, and then exhale slowly downward through your secret chakra, releasing the air, subtle air, and unwanted energy. Notice how you feel in your secret chakra.

5. Take a moment to notice how your whole central channel and your five chakras feel more open.

6. You will now do a movement to connect to your pervasive breath energy through your central channel and your whole body. Exhale all your stale air while contracting yourself into a curled sitting position. Notice how you feel almost devoid of air, and inhale smoothly through your side channels, continuing to guide your breath filling your central channel. Slowly stretch your body wide open to receive the air, feeling your air and energy expanding throughout your body and reaching the tips of your fingers through your arms, reaching your toes through your legs, and expanding into every sense organ in your head. Stay in that expansive sensation, comfortably holding your breath and energy. Exhale downward through your central channel, up your side channels, and out

your nostrils while you feel your subtle breath and energy releasing through all your pores. You can stay seated or let yourself fall backward. Then, remain in that position for a few moments.

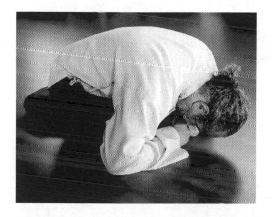

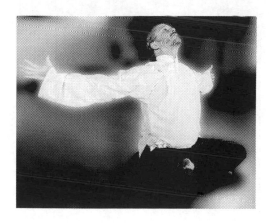

7. Assuming the cross-legged position and, if possible, the five-point meditation posture, continue feeling fully open and relaxed, with your focus directed throughout your entire body. Allow your breath-energy to permeate your body and beyond into the space around you.

8. Directly observe the changes in each of the chakras without engaging your intellect. Rest for a few moments with a meditative quality as you get ready to incorporate the magical movements.

CHAPTER 2

The Tibetan Yoga Movements from the *Instructions of the A*

HERE WE ARRIVE AT THE actual yogic movements of the Ligmincha Yoga of *Instructions of the A*.[1] In the previous steps, you learned about the importance of intention, having the proper body posture and breathings for this practice, and understanding and guiding your breath through your inner channels. Now you are ready to incorporate the magical movements. These practices involve breath retention for significant periods of time, therefore anyone with a physical, emotional, or psychological medical condition should consult with their physician before engaging in these practices.

There is one foundational movement (*ngondro* in Tibetan) and fifteen principal movements. The principal movements are divided into five sets of three movements each, with each set representing one of the five breath-energies.

Step 4: Incorporating the Movements

The Foundational Movement

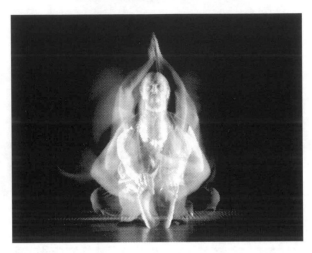

The foundational movement sets in motion the intention to connect to yourself and to benefit all beings as you energetically massage all your body and release the obstacles within yourself and all beings.

One of the most inspiring aspects of this practice is that we start with the intention of relieving not only our own suffering, but also that of all sentient beings. As you begin this movement, your hands will be at your heart to summon all your own sufferings and misdeeds along with those of all sentient beings in order to transform them and connect more deeply to the space of your own being that we call the "inner home."

1. Sit cross-legged, if possible, and place your hands in the *vajra* fist (see photo), with your right hand fisted on top of the left and both hands touching your *heart center,* the energetic center of your body-energy-mind system. Connect with your intention to relieve the suffering of yourself and others.

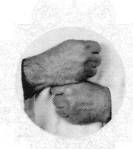

2. Sound *Hung* (pronounced hoong) seven times to call
    all suffering and misdeeds from all sentient beings,
    including yourself, visualizing them being attracted
    to a white *Hung*, or simply a white sphere of light at
    your navel chakra. The white light helps transform
    and "digest" those obstacles in the space of your
    navel chakra.

3. Inhale pervasively, letting the breath nurture your
    whole body. Holding your breath, extend your legs
    parallel to each other in front of you, use your hands
    to massage all parts of your body from head, to torso,
    to arms, to legs, and finally bring your hands toward
    your toes and hold them if possible. Keep holding
    your breath as you reach forward and internally
    connect with all the obstacles of yourself and others.

4. Shake all four limbs, and bend your knees, lightly
    stomping your feet on the floor and shaking your
    arms in the air. Imagine yourself stirring and clearing
    all those obstacles, and exhale thoroughly through
    your nose, followed by your mouth, while uttering
    the sounds *ha* and *phat*. Return to the cross-legged
    position or assume the five-point posture, feeling
    the rhythm of your breath and reconnecting to your
    meditative state.

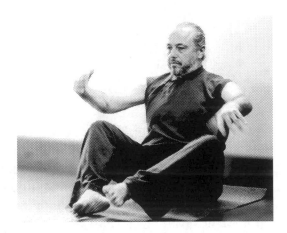

This last step is also the concluding motion for all 15 principal movements that follow. You can do it in a sitting or standing posture.

Texts and teachers emphasize the importance of remembering to do this concluding motion at the end of each Tibetan yoga movement, as it internally stirs all the afflictions, obstacles, and obscurations of not just yourself, but all beings. This enacts your intention to expel obstacles and reconnect to your meditative state and inner home.

The use of the sounds *ha* and *phat* are unique to the Tibetan yoga of the Bon tradition. *Ha* is used to help clear illnesses and obstacles, and *phat* helps cut through the elaborations of your mind and get you more in touch with the space within and awareness of your inner home.

You are, of course, not expected to be totally clear of obstacles after one session. Rather, think of this as a process, like pouring clean water into the dirty bottle of your mind-energy-body system, stirring it, and pouring the water back out. The more you do this, the cleaner the bottle will be. Performing these Tibetan yoga movements has a cumulative effect, cleansing you and helping you become more familiar with and more settled in your meditative state and connected with the natural state of your mind (i.e., your inner home), which is represented by the letter *A* in the Tibetan yoga of *Instructions of the A*.

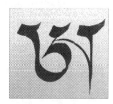

The Fifteen Principal Magical Movements

I find it particularly poignant that the principal movements of the Tibetan yoga of *Instructions of the A* start with a focus on your heart center. This practice starts at the heart, then goes to the head, then down to the navel, and finally down to reengage the whole body and energy system. Other Tibetan yoga practices usually start with the head and go down or start at the bottom and go up.

In the foundational movement, you started by touching your heart and then used your whole energetic body through your pervasive breath. By breathing into your central channel and holding your breath as you massaged your whole body, you cleared the major obstacles of your body, energy, and mind. You have released some pains or tensions. You felt the breath-energy flowing better through your body and your mind becoming a little more calm and focused.

The principal movements are designed to clear the obstacles of your upper torso, head, abdomen, lower torso and legs, in that order. Each set of three principal movements clears one of the five parts of the body and focuses on a different chakra or chakras or in the whole central channel, and on a different breath-energy. Each breath-energy correlates with one of the five elements, and in this way, you balance your mind-energy-body system—achieving the goal of Tibetan medicine—as well as balancing yourself and your environment, the microcòsm and macrocosm, which is the goal of yoga.

Now, bring your attention to the center of your central channel: your heart chakra.

SET 1: UPPER-TORSO PURIFICATION

Body part: Torso
Chakra: Heart
Breath-energy: Life force
Element: Space

For the three movements of the **Upper-Torso Purification,** begin by focusing on your heart center. As you connect with your **life-force** breath-energy, you will feel the openness of your heart chakra, supported by the space element.

Each movement in this set of three upper-torso purification movements begins with inhaling through your nostrils and welcoming and guiding your breath by visualizing it following your side channels to reach your central channel. As your breath-energy enters your central channel at the junction of the three channels (four fingers below your navel), guide it up your central channel and hold it at your heart chakra. Feel that hold (without locking) and maintain it throughout the movement as you hold your breath like nectar in a vase, (i.e., keeping the breath's nutrients in your body).

At the conclusion of each of these three movements, guide your breath down your central channel to the junction of the three channels and up the side channels and then release it through your nostrils. The subtle exhalation is released through your heart chakra itself, almost as if the chakra is a valve releasing its air along with your energetic and emotionally charged obstacles.

After doing one repetition of each of the three upper-torso purification movements, come back to the cross-legged position or five-point posture. Notice how you feel in your heart chakra, supported by the space element. Rest your mind as you keep softly guiding your breath from your nose into your heart chakra and back out through your nose.

*Principal Movement #1: Stretching the Bow to Shoot an Arrow
(Da pen zhu pen)*

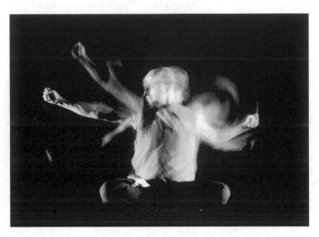

1. Sit in the cross-legged position with your hands resting on your lap in the equipoise position—palms up, left hand over right, thumbs at the bases of your ring fingers. Inhale into your heart chakra and hold your breath there for a moment to feel your life-force breath-energy. Keep holding it throughout the movement. If you can't hold your breath throughout the whole movement, you can do less repetitions or reinhale when needed.

2. Holding your breath, form both hands into loose fists, as if you are holding a bow and about to extend its string to shoot an arrow. Extend the left arm diagonally to the left side and then skyward. Raise your right arm and pull it back three times, as if you are pulling back the string on the bow. Do the movement at a speed at which you can feel the stretching of your body and of the air in your heart

chakra. Then do the movement three times while aiming downward at the earth and three times while aiming level to the horizon.

3. On the right side, as you maintain your focus and keep holding the breath in your heart chakra, repeat the movements, extending your right arm and pulling back with the left three times toward the sky, the earth, and the horizon. Each time you pull back the string, feel the heart chakra space slowly expanding and the life-force breath-energy helping to loosen whatever obstacles of body, energy, and mind you are storing.

4. After you finish stretching the bow on both sides, perform the concluding motion: Shake and stir your arms and legs to help release the obstacles you have loosened up within yourself and within all sentient beings.

5. Exhale through your nose, then make the sounds *ha* and *phat* to assist in thoroughly cleansing the obstacles from your heart chakra and with the intention of extending the cleansing to all sentient beings.

6. After exhaling, abide in that more open, relaxed state of mind, which is supported by the slight exhaustion of your body.

7. Remain in that state of mind, noticing your breath and settling more into the meditative *A* state of mind.

8. Continue to focus on your heart chakra, which may have a greater sense of openness supported by the space element, and make sure your mind is guiding your breath as you continue to the next movement.

Principal Movement #2: Dropping a Stone from Your Waist
(Ke pa do gyur)

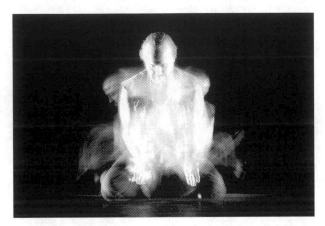

1. Sit in the cross-legged position with your hands resting on your lap in the equipoise position. Inhale into your heart chakra and hold your breath there for a moment. Bring your elbows to your waist and your arms to the front, and then bend forward from the waist. Imagine that you are lifting a large stone with both hands in front of you.

2. Grab the stone, rotate your torso to the right and place the stone on the floor at your right side. Then return to the center position. Repeat the movement two more times, from the center to the right, as if there are three different stones to move.

3. While continuing to hold your breath at your heart chakra, move the stone from the center to your left side, then return to the center, three times.

4. Still holding your breath at your heart chakra, pick up and hold out the stone in front of you, rolling slightly forward on your legs to drop the stone farther in front of you. Then return to the original position. Repeat this movement two more times.

5. Perform the concluding motion: Shake and stir your arms and legs so you can feel the obstacles the movements have loosened up within you being released, together with those of all sentient beings.

6. Exhale through your nose, and then make the sounds *ha* and *phat* to assist in thoroughly cleansing the obstacles from your heart chakra and with the intention of extending the cleansing to all sentient beings.

7. After exhaling, abide in that more open, relaxed state of mind, which is supported by the slight exhaustion of your body.

8. Remain in that state of mind, noticing your breath and settling more into that meditative, or *A*, state of mind.

9. Continue to focus on your heart chakra, making sure your mind is guiding your breath, as you continue to the next movement.

Principal Movement #3: Swimmer's Stroke (Kyal pa kyal chap)

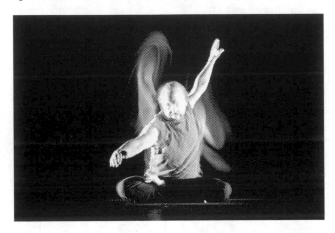

1. Sit in the cross-legged position with your hands resting on your lap in the equipoise position. Inhale into your heart chakra and hold your breath there for a moment. Bend slightly forward.

2. Alternate moving your arms as if you are swimming using the freestyle stroke. Do this for a total of 21 strokes, starting with your right arm, so your right arm will make 11 strokes and your left will make 10. Feel how the movement expands your chest area and the air in your heart chakra.

3. Perform the concluding motion: Shake and stir your arms and legs so you can feel the obstacles the stretches have loosened up within you being released, along with those of all sentient beings.

4. Exhale through your nose, then make the sounds *ha* and *phat* to assist in thoroughly cleansing the obstacles from your heart chakra and with

the intention of extending the cleansing to all
sentient beings.

5. After exhaling, abide in that more open, relaxed state
    of mind, which is supported by the slight exhaustion
    of your body.

6. Remain in that state of mind, noticing your breath
    and settling more into that meditative, or *A*,
    state of mind.

Benefits of the Upper-Torso Purification movements

These three Upper-Torso Purification movements expand your
chest in different ways. Notice the physical expansion in your
body, particularly in your heart and upper torso area, and how
the slight exhaustion helps your mind settle at your heart center.
Energetically, having worked with the life-force breath-energy, you
may feel a nourishing of your mind-heart area. This is important,
as it enables you to abide with more awareness at the spaciousness
of your heart center supported by the space element. When your
mind-heart is more calm and open, you are able to maintain a
meditative state, with less engagement of your conceptual mind.

At MD Anderson, we begin our meditation and Tibetan yoga
sessions with the Connecting with Your Heart meditation (page
5). In fact, if you want to train your mind to be less of a monkey
mind and more settled in your mind-heart energetic center, you
can start with the Connecting with Your Heart meditation and
then follow with these principal movements of the Upper-Torso
Purification to abide longer there. This familiarization with your
mind-heart energetic center can be a great foundation as you continue to practice this yoga.

SET 2: HEAD PURIFICATION

Body part: Head
Chakra: Throat and crown
Breath-energy: Upward moving
Element: Earth

For the three movements of the **Head Purification**, begin by focusing on your throat chakra and connecting with the **upward-moving** breath-energy. At the end of each movement, exhale and release obstacles through your crown chakra while maintaining a sense of grounding and embodiment at your throat chakra, which connects to the support of the earth element.

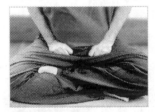 For the movements in this set, start in the cross-legged seated position, with your hands forming *vajra* fists by placing your thumbs at the base of your ring fingers and making a fist. Then press slightly at your inguinal crease (where the leg begins below the torso). Extend your arms to lengthen and straighten your torso and then slightly relax your shoulders.

Each movement begins with inhaling through both nostrils and welcoming and guiding your breath by visualizing it following your side channels. As your breath-energy enters your central channel at the junction, guide it up your central channel and hold it at your throat chakra. In that hold, the throat stays soft and relaxed (without a *bandha* or lock), and you can feel the ascending quality of your upward-moving breath-energy, supported by the movement of your head.

At the conclusion of each of these head-purification movements, focus on the subtle exhalation released upward through your crown chakra, releasing its air along with your energetic and emotionally charged obstacles. Feel the support of the earth element at your throat chakra as you remain grounded, guiding your subtle breath down your central channel to the junction of the three channels and up the side channels, and then releasing your physical breath through your nostrils.

After doing all three of the head-purification movements one time, come back to the cross-legged position or five-point posture. Notice how you feel in your throat and crown chakras and rest your mind in that sense of openness and stability in your meditative, or *A*, state of mind.

Principal Movement #4: Bending the Neck (Ke kyok)

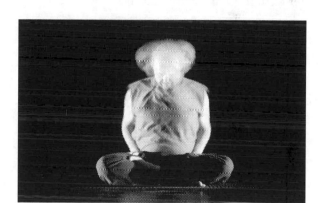

1. Sit in the cross-legged position with your hands in vajra fists at your inguinal crease. Inhale into your throat chakra and hold your breath there for a moment.

2. Continue to hold your breath as you bend your head and neck as far as it can go but without straining forward, backward, to the right, and to the left, traveling through the center position each time and feeling the breath energy moving upward. Repeat two more times.

3. Perform the concluding motion: Shake and stir your arms and legs so you can feel the obstacles the movements have loosened up within you being released, together with those of all sentient beings.

4. Exhale through your crown chakra and your nostrils, and then make the sounds *ha* and *phat* to aid in thoroughly cleansing the obstacles from your throat and crown chakras and with the intention of extending the cleansing to all sentient beings.

5. After exhaling, abide in that more open and relaxed meditative, or *A*, state of mind, supported by a slight sense of decongestion in your head.

6. Continue to focus on your throat and crown chakras, making sure your mind is guiding your breath as you continue to the next movement.

Principal Movement #5: Bouncing the Hair-Knot (Ral gyur)

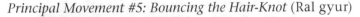

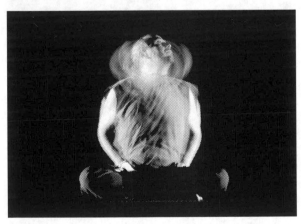

1. Sit in the cross-legged position with your hands in *vajra* fists at your inguinal crease. Inhale into your throat chakra and hold your breath there for a moment.

2. Continue to hold your breath as you bend your head slightly forward and to your right, and then swing your head to your front left to gain momentum. Toss your head backward and to your right, as if moving a hair topknot to your right, as you feel your breath energy moving upward. Return to the starting position and repeat this action two more times.

3. In the same way described in Step 2, bend your head slightly forward and then to your left, and then swing it to your front right to gain momentum. Toss your head backward and to your left, as if moving a hair topknot to the left, as you feel your breath-energy moving upward and backward to the left. Return to the starting position and repeat this action two more times.

4. Toss your head—or "topknot"—straight from front to back, bending your head forward and then swinging it backward, for a total of three times, feeling your breath-energy moving upward with each movement.

5. Perform the concluding motion: Shake and stir your arms and legs so you can feel the obstacles the movements have loosened up within you being released, together with those of all sentient beings.

6. Exhale through your crown chakra and your nostrils, and then make the sounds *ha* and *phat* to assist in thoroughly cleansing the obstacles from your throat and crown chakras and with the intention of extending the cleansing to all sentient beings.

7. After exhaling, abide in that more open and relaxed meditative, or *A*, state of mind, supported by a slight sense of decongestion in your head.

8. Continue to focus on your throat and crown chakras, making sure that your mind is guiding your breath as you continue to the next movement.

Principal Movement #6: Rolling the Head (Go ril)

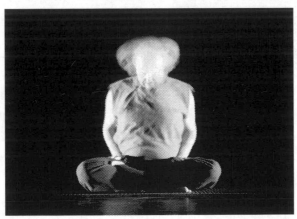

1. Sit in the cross-legged position with your hands in *vajra* fists at your inguinal crease. Inhale into your throat chakra and hold your breath there for a moment.

2. Continue to hold your breath as you roll your head and neck counterclockwise three times. Repeat in the clockwise direction three times. Throughout both motions, feel your breath-energy moving upward.

3. Perform the concluding motion: Shake and stir your arms and legs so you can feel the obstacles the movements have loosened up within you being released, together with those of all sentient beings.

4. Exhale through your crown chakra and your nostrils, then make the sounds *hu* and *phat* to assist in thoroughly cleansing the obstacles from your throat and crown chakras and with the intention of extending the cleansing to all sentient beings.

5. After exhaling, abide in that more open and relaxed meditative, or *A*, state of mind, supported by a slight sense of decongestion in your head.

Benefits of the head-purification movements

With these three head-purification movements, you use your upward-moving breath-energy to clear your head and sense organs. Notice the clearing and decongestion of your head, helping you release conceptual grasping and relax more into your meditative, or *A*, state of mind. You may feel more open in your crown chakra, as well as more settled in your throat chakra, supported by the earth element.

SET 3: BODY PURIFICATION

Body part: Body, and especially abdomen
Chakra: Navel
Breath-energy: Fire-like
Element: Fire

In the three movements of **Body Purification**, you will bring the **fire-like** breath-energy into your navel chakra with the support of the fire element.

Each movement in this set begins with inhaling through your nostrils and welcoming and guiding your breath by visualizing it following your side channels. As your breath-energy enters your central channel at the junction, guide it up to your navel chakra. Hold your breath-energy by pulling your stomach inward toward your spine, which is called "bringing the ocean to the rocks." Maintain this hold throughout each of these three movements.

At the conclusion of each movement, guide your breath down your central channel to the junction and up the side channels, then release it through your nostrils. Release the hold and the subtle exhalation through your navel chakra, almost as if the chakra were a valve releasing air along with your energetic and emotionally charged obstacles.

After doing all three body-purification movements one time, come back to the cross-legged position or five-point posture. Notice how you feel in your navel chakra. You may feel more warmth, supported by the fire element. Rest your mind in that sense of awareness.

The third movement of this set is done standing up, and I will tell you how to do the concluding movement in the standing posture below.

Principal Movement #7: Striking the Tops of the Shoulders
(Pung go dek)

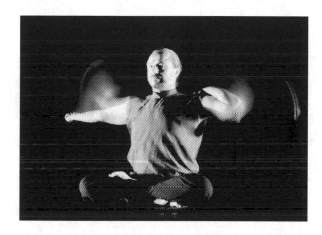

1. Sit cross-legged. Inhale, bring "the ocean to the rocks," and extend your arms straight out to both sides with your elbows pointing downward. Form *vajra* fists with the palms of your hands facing upward.

2. Continue holding your breath and your fists as you bend your right elbow and strike your right shoulder with the knuckles of your right hand. As you extend your right arm again, use your left fist to strike your left shoulder. Alternate this striking movement for 9 strikes on each side (for a total of 18 strikes).

3. Perform the concluding motion: Shake and stir your arms and legs so you can feel the obstacles the movements have loosened up within you being released, together with those of all sentient beings.

4. Exhale through your nose, then make the sounds *ha* and *phat* as you release the retention of the ocean to the rocks to assist in thoroughly cleansing the obstacles from your navel chakra and with the intention of extending the cleansing to all sentient beings.

5. After exhaling, abide in that more open and relaxed meditative, or *A*, state of mind, supported by a slight sense of warmth around your navel.

6. Continue to focus on your navel chakra, making sure your mind is guiding your breath as you continue to the next movement.

Principal Movement #8: Liberating the Orifices (Bu ka nam dröl)

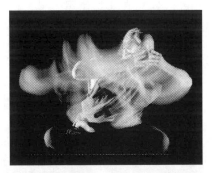

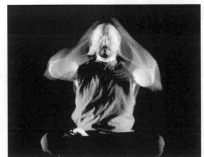
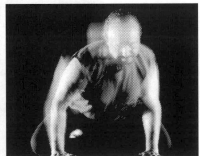

1. Sit in the cross-legged position. Inhale, bring "the ocean to the rocks," and raise your hands to your face and cover each ear canal with the thumb of the corresponding hand. Cover each eyelid with the corresponding index finger, press your nostrils closed with your middle fingers, and place your ring fingers above your mouth and your pinky fingers below your mouth to hold your mouth shut.

2. Continue holding your breath as you rotate your torso in a movement called "soaring over the shoulders" or "soaring with your torso." Guided by your left shoulder, rotate your torso three times counterclockwise, and then, guided by your right shoulder, rotate your torso three times clockwise, always keeping your focus at your navel.

3. Keeping your thumbs on your ears, wipe your fingers and palms downward over your face—eyes and cheeks—three times. Remove your hands.

4. While still holding your breath, extend your left arm to the front, and then quickly sweep your right hand down your left arm, from the shoulder to the hand, three times. Then repeat the motion, sweeping your left hand down your right arm, three times.

5. Roll up onto your knees and place both hands on the floor in front of you. Vigorously shake your torso from side to side three times.

6. Perform the concluding motion: Shake and stir your arms and legs so you can feel the obstacles the movements have loosened up within you being released, together with those of all sentient beings.

7. Exhale through your nose, then make the sounds *ha* and *phat* as you release the retention of the ocean to the rocks to assist in thoroughly cleansing the obstacles from your navel chakra and with the intention of extending the cleansing to all sentient beings.

8. After exhaling, abide in that more open and relaxed meditative, or *A*, state of mind, supported by a slight sense of warmth at your navel.

9. Continue to focus on your navel chakra, making sure your mind is guiding your breath as you continue to the next movement.

Principal Movement #9: Throwing the Lasso (Zhak pa ma)

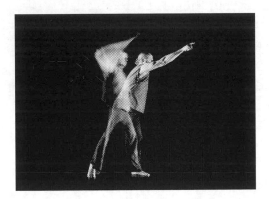

1. Stand up. Step forward one stride with your left leg. Facing straight ahead, place your hands on your hips.

2. While keeping your elbow bent, inhale, bring "the ocean to the rocks," and pull your right arm to the back, and then bring it to the side and swing a couple

of times like you are twirling a lasso. Then throw your arm forward, as if you are throwing a lasso. When you throw the lasso across your front, rotate your torso to the left to make the release stronger. Repeat, throwing the lasso two more times.

3. While continuing to hold your breath, reverse the positions of your legs and throw the lasso three times with your left hand.

4. Perform the concluding motion from the standing posture: Jump a couple of times, and then shake and stir your arms and legs so you can feel the obstacles the movements have loosened up within you being released, together with those of all sentient beings.

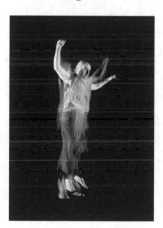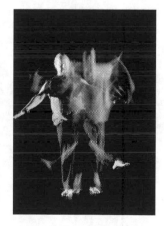

5. Exhale through your nose, then make the sounds *ha* and *phat* as you release the retention of the ocean to the rocks to assist in thoroughly cleansing the obstacles from your navel chakra and with the intention of extending the cleansing to all sentient beings.

6. After exhaling, return to the cross-legged position or five-point posture and abide in that more open and relaxed meditative, or *A*, state of mind, supported by a slight sense of warmth at your navel.

Benefits of the Body-Purification Movements

With this set of body-purification movements, you clear the area around your navel in different ways. You will notice some physical warmth in your body, particularly in your abdominal area, and that the slight exhaustion has helped your mind to settle. Energetically, the fire-like breath-energy may make you feel an energetic nourishing and warmth in the areas of your navel and abdomen. This is important, because this warmth, supported by the fire element, can help you be more comfortable, relaxed, and supported in your meditative state of *A*. This warmth also cultivates your creativity.

SET 4: LOWER-TORSO PURIFICATION

Body part: Lower torso
Chakra: Secret
Breath-energy: Downward-moving and clearing
Element: Water

With the three movements of the **Lower-Torso Purification**, you bring the **downward-moving and clearing** breath-energy into your secret chakra (at your perineum, the place between your genitals and your anus), where you will apply the "basket hold" of lifting your pelvic floor, feeling the support of the water element.

Each movement in this set begins with inhaling through your nostrils and welcoming and guiding your breath by visualizing it following your side channels. As your breath-energy enters the base of your central channel, hold it in your secret chakra by bringing your pelvic floor up with the basket hold—tightening the anal sphincter and lifting the whole pelvic floor—similar to Kegel exercises. Maintain this hold throughout each of these three movements.

At the conclusion of each of the lower-torso purification movements, guide your breath from your central channel and up the side channels, and then release it through your nostrils. The subtle exhalation is released through your secret chakra itself, releasing the basket hold, and almost as if the chakra is a valve releasing its air downward along with your energetic and emotionally charged obstacles, supported by the comfort of the water element.

After doing all three lower-torso purification movements one time, return to the cross-legged position or five-point posture. Notice how you feel in your secret chakra. You may feel comfort from the support of the water element. Rest your mind in that sense of comfortable awareness.

Principal Movement #10: Rotating in the Dorje Posture
(Tra pü ma)

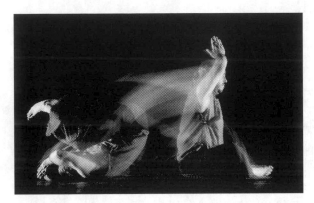

1. Sit in the *dorje* pose, with the soles of your feet touching each other, your bent arms extended overhead, and your palms touching.

2. Inhale into your secret chakra with the basket hold, and roll forward and then backward a total of nine times.

3. Perform the concluding motion either sitting or standing: Shake and stir your arms and legs so you can feel the obstacles the movements have loosened up within you being released, together with those of all sentient beings.

4. Exhale through your nose, then make the sounds *ha* and *phat* as you release the basket retention to assist in thoroughly cleansing the obstacles from your secret chakra and with the intention of extending the cleansing to all sentient beings.

5. After exhaling, assume the cross-legged position. Notice how you feel in your secret chakra. You may feel comfort from the support of the water element. Rest your mind in that sense of comfortable awareness and abide in that more open and relaxed meditative, or *A*, state of mind.

6. Continue to focus on your secret chakra, making sure your mind is guiding your breath as you continue to the next movement.

Principal Movement #11: Four [Limbs] Kicking (Zhi tra ma)

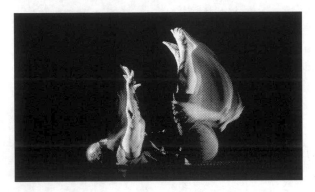

1. Inhale with the basket hold as you lie on your back and reach your arms and legs up toward the sky.

2. Simultaneously bend and bring your arms and legs in toward your body and then thrust them skyward. Repeat this bringing in and thrusting out eight more times.

3. Perform the concluding motion: Shake and stir your arms and legs so you can feel the obstacles the movements have loosened up within you being released, together with those of all sentient beings.

4. Exhale through your nose, then make the sounds *ha* and *phat* as you release the basket retention to assist in thoroughly cleansing the obstacles from your secret chakra and with the intention of extending the cleansing to all sentient beings.

5. After exhaling, assume the cross-legged position. Notice how you feel in your secret chakra. You may feel comfort from the support of the water element. Rest your mind in that sense of comfortable awareness and abide in that more open and relaxed meditative or *A*, state of mind.

6. Continue to focus on your secret chakra, making sure your mind is guiding your breath as you continue to the next movement.

*Principal Movement #12: Generating the Powerful Tigle*s (Tigle top gye)

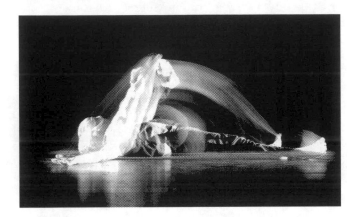

1. Inhale with the basket hold and lie on your back with your arms out to your sides and your legs spread apart.

2. Visualize a yellow bowstring between your feet (held by the big toes). It is holding a fire arrow pointing toward your body, with its tip directed at your secret chakra.

3. Sound a long *hung* and imagine all substantial obstacles as spheres—*tigles*—that are accumulating in the arrowhead as the bowstring becomes increasingly taut.

4. Sound a strong *phat* and quickly bend your legs, bring them to your stomach, and then grab them with your hands as you imagine the released arrow coursing through your central channel, exiting through your crown chakra, and releasing all your tigles into space, where they dissolve. Rest for a moment in that sense of dissolution.

5. Inhale again into your secret chakra with the basket hold and do the concluding motion sitting or standing: Shake and stir your arms and legs so you can feel the obstacles the movements have loosened up within you being released, together with those of all sentient beings.

6. Exhale through your nose, and then make the sounds *ha* and *phat* as you release the basket retention to assist in thoroughly cleansing the obstacles from your secret chakra and with the intention of extending the cleansing to all sentient beings.

7. After exhaling, assume the cross-legged position or five-point posture. Notice how you feel in your secret chakra. You may feel comfort from the support of the water element. Rest your mind in that sense of comfortable awareness and abide in that more open and relaxed meditative, or *A*, state of mind.

Benefits of the Lower-Torso Purification Movements

With this set of lower-torso purification movements, you clear your secret chakra in different ways. Notice now how you feel there, including your physical comfort, particularly in your lower-torso, and how the slight exhaustion helps your mind to settle. Energetically, having worked with the downward-moving and clearing breath-energy, you may feel a sense of release and comfort in your secret chakra and lower-torso, supported by the water element. This is important, because this comfort can help you be more at ease, relaxed, and supported in your meditative state of *A*.

SET 5: LEG PURIFICATION

Body part: Legs, and whole body
Subtle body: Central channel
Breath-energy: Pervasive
Element: Air

The three movements of **Leg Purification** are performed standing. In each movement, there is a jump that aids the distribution throughout your body of the **pervasive** breath-energy with the support of the air, or wind, element.

Each movement in this set begins by standing and inhaling through your nostrils and welcoming and guiding your breath by visualizing it following your side channels. You will then bring your breath-energy into your whole central channel and hold it softly in what is called "neutral retention" (without *bandha*, or lock), a sense of focusing on your central channel to support the pervasive breath-energy's expansion throughout your body.

At the conclusion of each leg-purification movement, guide your breath from your central channel and up the side channels, and then release it through your nostrils. The subtle exhalation is released through every pore of your body, taking with it your energetic and emotionally charged obstacles, supported by the force of the wind, or air, element.

After doing all of the leg-purification movements one time, assume the cross-legged position or five-point posture. Notice how you feel in your central channel and your whole body. You may feel a sense of expansion and an inner flexibility, supported by the air element. Rest your mind in that sense of expansive awareness.

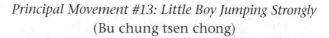

Principal Movement #13: Little Boy Jumping Strongly
(Bu chung tsen chong)

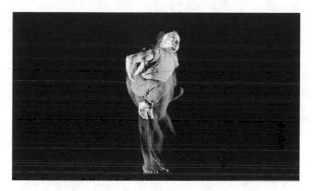

1.   Stand with your feet together and your hands on your hips.

2.   Inhale into your central channel and make nine small vertical jumps, followed by nine larger vertical jumps—allowing your knees to bend as needed—feeling how the jumps aid in the expansion of the pervasive breath-energy throughout your body and the clearing of obstacles.

3.   Perform the concluding motion from the standing posture: Jump a couple of times, and then shake and stir your arms and legs so you can feel the obstacles the movements have loosened up within you being released, together with those of all sentient beings.

4.   Exhale through your nose, then make the sounds *ha* and *phat* as you feel a sense of release from every pore of your body, assisting in thoroughly cleansing

the obstacles from your central channel and your whole body and with the intention of extending the cleansing to all sentient beings.

5. After exhaling, assume the cross-legged position. Notice how you feel in your central channel and whole body, supported by the pervasive energy-breath and the air element. Abide and rest in that more open and relaxed meditative, or *A*, state of mind, supported by a slight sense of expansiveness and flexibility in your whole body.

6. Continue to focus on your central channel and breathe pervasively, making sure your mind is guiding your breath as you continue to the next movement.

Principal Movement #14: Elephant Kicking Back and Forth
(Lang chen nga tra chi tra)

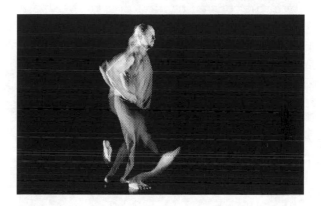

1. Stand with your right foot in front of your left and with your hands on your hips. Inhale into your central channel as you bring your weight on your left foot and you lift your right foot with a slight kick forward. Then hop back on your right foot, swinging back your left foot. As you continue to hold your breath, repeat this back-and-forth movement, kicking with your right foot forward and swinging back your left a total of nine times.

2. While still holding your breath, bring your left foot in front of your right. Then bring your weight on your right foot, "kick" forward with the left, and then with the weight forward on your left foot, swing your right foot backward. Continue performing the movement, kicking forward with your left foot and swinging back with your right foot for a total of nine times. Feel how the jumping supports the pervasive

breath energy's expansion throughout and clearing the obstacles from your whole body.

3. Perform the concluding motion from the standing posture: Jump a couple of times, and then shake and stir your arms and legs so you can feel the obstacles the movements have loosened up within you being released, together with those of all sentient beings.

4. Exhale through your nose, then make the sounds *ha* and *phat* as you feel a sense of release from every pore, assisting in thoroughly cleansing the obstacles from your central channel and your whole body and with the intention of extending the cleansing to all sentient beings.

5. After exhaling, assume the cross-legged position. Notice how you feel in your central channel and whole body. You may feel a sense of expansion and inner flexibility, supported by the air element. Abide and rest in that more open and relaxed meditative, or *A*, state of mind, supported by a slight sense of expansiveness and flexibility in your whole body.

6. Continue to focus on your central channel and breathe pervasively, making sure your mind is guiding your breath as you continue to the next movement.

Principal Movement #15: Placing the Sole of the Foot at the Knee
(Pu mor til jok)

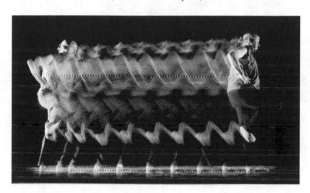

1. Inhale into your central channel as you stand on your left foot and place the sole of your right foot against your left leg at the side of your knee. Hop forward nine times.

2. Keep holding your breath pervasively, as you turn and reverse the position, standing on your right leg and placing the sole of your left foot against your right leg at the side of your knee. Hop forward nine times. Feel how the jumps support the pervasive breath-energy's expansion throughout and the clearing of obstacles from your whole body.

3. Perform the concluding motion from the standing posture: Jump a couple of times, and then shake and stir your arms and legs so you can feel the obstacles

the movements have loosened up within you being released, together with those of all sentient beings.

4. Exhale through your nose, and then make the sounds *ha* and *phat* as you feel a sense of release from every pore, assisting in thoroughly cleansing the obstacles from your central channel and your whole body and with the intention of extending the cleansing to all sentient beings.

5. After exhaling, assume the cross-legged position or five-point posture. Notice how you feel in your central channel and whole body. You may feel a sense of expansion and inner flexibility, supported by the air element. Abide and rest in that more open and relaxed meditative, or *A*, state of mind, supported by a slight sense of expansiveness and flexibility in your whole body.

Benefits of the Leg-Purification Movements

With each of these three leg-purification movements, you clear the obstacles from your legs, and by jumping, you clear the obstacles from your whole body. Notice now how you feel in your whole body physically and how the sense of exhaustion helps your mind to settle. Energetically, after working with your pervasive breath-energy, you may feel greater flexibility in your legs and expansion from your central channel to your whole body, supported by your pervasive breath-energy and the air element. This is important, because this expansion and flexibility can help you feel more at ease and supported to stay longer in your meditative state of *A*.

Concluding Your Session

You now have cleared all five parts of your body and your five chakras, balancing your five breath-energies. Come back to the five-point posture or lie down in corpse pose, or *shavasana*. Remain relaxed but with open awareness for as long as the experience remains fresh. This is an important part of the practice, so try not to fall asleep. Instead, enjoy the benefits of all the movements and the exhaustion so you can be more connected to your natural state of mind, your meditative state of A. *That is the magic!*

If you are lying down, now sit up and assume the five-point posture. Take a few moments to gradually notice how you feel in each of your five chakras and your whole central channel. Allow your body to support you in connecting with and staying in your meditative A state of mind.

Step 5: Share the Benefits of Your Practice

In order to share the benefits of your practice, you can start by feeling grateful to your teachers and their teachings and to yourself for having practiced, and then share the good sensations you're feeling with others. You may want to share with those who you know are suffering or going through difficult moments, or you may just share this practice with everyone for a sense of well-being for all. It is important to feel you can include all sentient beings in your sharing. The Tibetan tradition calls this the dedication of one's practice, with the metaphor that what we share is like nectar that we pour into the ocean, and there is enough for everyone, including yourself. Those benefits will be there until the ocean dries up. If you do not share your good sensations, if you put the benefits in your own little cup, in a moment of thirst, or anger, or greed, they are gone. So make sure you take a moment to share the benefits of your practice with others as much as you do with yourself.

CHAPTER 3

A Brief History of
the Bon Tibetan Yoga

The Himalayan traditions are rich in mind-body practices used for spiritual development in the quest for enlightenment and for physical and emotional well-being. Within the Tibetan tradition, numerous yogic practices that have been practiced for centuries in Tibet, Nepal, and India have migrated to other countries. The globalization that took place in the 20th century allowed many of these practices to take root in the West.

The yogas of this book come from the ancient Tibetan Bon tradition, and, thanks to teachers like His Holiness Lungtok Tenpai Nyima and Yongdzin Tenzin Namdak, they migrated to India and Nepal, and then arrived in the United States and other Western countries. They were preserved not only in texts, but also in practice, both in monasteries and in yogic communities. As with many yogic traditions, it is very important to know that there is a lineage of teachings passing from master to disciple, from teacher to student. In this chapter, I will provide you with a brief history of the Tibetan Yoga of *Instructions of the A* so you can know their origin and key teachers and understand why it is only recently that they are being introduced in the West and becoming more available to you.

Early Teachers and Masters

Gongdzo Ritro Chenpo and Drogon Lodro were two important 11th-century masters in the Bon tradition, particularly with regard to the *Instructions of the A*. Gongdzo Ritro Chenpo compiled the teachings that became the whole text of *Instructions of the A*,[1] and Drogon Lodro compiled the Tibetan yoga chapter within that text. In that chapter, Drogon Lodro mentions 41 movements, 1 foundational (*ngondro*) and 40 principal, the latter of which are divided into the five body groups—7 movements for the upper torso, 6 for the head, 11 for the body, 9 for the lower torso and 7 for the legs.

In the 13th century, the great Bon master and scholar Dru Gyalwa Yungdrung was known for compiling teachings and creating manuals so practitioners could follow the teachings more easily and, more important, perform the practices and understand their experiences.

In his manual for the *Instructions of the A*, Dru Gyalwa Yungdrung included the chapter on Tibetan yoga, condensing the 40 magical movements into 16—1 foundational and 15 principal—but he did not divide them into the five different parts of the body, as Drogon Lodro's original text did.

Shardza Tashi Gyaltsen Rinpoche

Shardza Tashi Gyaltsen deserves a category of his own. He lived in the eastern Tibetan province of Kham in the late-19th and early

20th centuries and was one of the most prominent Tibetan yogic figures. In 1934, he attained the rainbow body, which the tradition holds is a sign of the highest contemplative state. He was a great scholar and practitioner not only in Bon, but also in the nonsectarian tradition (*ri med*). He wrote commentaries on various texts, including some Tibetan yoga texts. For the *Yoga of the Instructions of the A*, his commentary has two parts, one on the 40 movements by Drogon Lodro and another on the 16 movements by Dru Gyalwa Yungdrung. Many of my teachers trained using Shardza's commentaries, and thanks to them, I received and practiced those teachings. Shardza was also the author of the manual for the 100-day Tibetan yoga retreat that I utilized for my training at Menri Monastery.

Since connecting to the Bon tradition and its Tibetan contemplative practices, I have felt inspired by Shardza's work and example, particularly by how Shardza helped transmit these practices beyond the limits of the Bon tradition as part of the nonsectarian movement, while still keeping their purity and power. In my first book, *Chöd Practice in the Bon Tradition*, I translated Shardza's commentary on that practice, and in my dissertation, I translated Shardza's commentary on the Tibetan yoga of *The Oral Transmission of Zhang Zhung*. Shardza's commentaries have been invaluable as I learn and practice the Tibetan Yoga of *Instructions of the A*, and when I trained following his retreat program. During a trip to Tibet in 2007, Tenzin Wangyal Rinpoche invited a yogi trained at Shardza's retreat center in the Kham region of Tibet to Lhasa, in Central Tibet, where we met and corroborated these teachings. This yogi, who was one of Shardza's direct students, showed us the way he had been trained in Shardza's lineage. I value the few hours we spent together like a rare and very precious jewel. Shardza has been an incredible example as a scholar and practitioner, and as a teacher who has inspired so many of his followers to the present day.

In the 1950s, with the changes during China's invasion and occupation of Tibet, Tibetan wisdom teachings became endangered, but thanks to teachers like Yongdzin Tenzin Namdak and His Holiness Lungtok Tenpai Nyima, they have been preserved in exile, in India, Nepal, and the West. It is hard not to have a soft heart and some tears when I think of the hardships they went through and how fortunate many of us are to have received teachings directly from them. From that place in my heart, I'll share some of their stories so you too can receive what they taught me.

Contemporary Masters

Yongdzin Tenzin Namdak Rinpoche, one of the most revered Tibetan teachers and indeed the most revered Bon teacher alive, was born in the Kham province of Tibet in 1926, and escaped in 1959, after the Chinese occupation, arriving safely (although with a bullet in his left knee) in Nepal and then India. Together with His Holiness Lungtok Tenpai Nyima, he was instrumental in maintaining the Bon teachings in exile, helping to found and construct Menri Monastery in India and Triten Norbutse in Nepal.

In 1991, Namkhai Norbu Rinpoche directed me to Yongdzin Tenzin Namdak, and since then I have had the great fortune of studying with him for over 25 years, including the teachings from the *Instructions of the A*. I first learned the Bon yoga in his Triten Norbutse Monastery in 1993 and then was able to ask him questions during the many years I was researching for and writing my Ph.D. dissertation. During my visits to Triten Norbutse, I was able to train with the yogic group and consult with Yongdzin Tenzin

Namdak almost daily. His clarity over the years, as well as the support of Khenpo Nyima Wangyal and Khenpo Tenpa Yungdrung, has been invaluable.

Yongdzin Tenzin Namdak has also been very supportive of my bringing these practices into medical settings. Before designing the first research study using Tibetan yoga for people with cancer, I consulted with him not only on the content, but also to ask his permission to bring these practices into a Western medical context. He kindly agreed, and whenever we met afterward, whether in Nepal, France, or the United States, he wanted to know more about how the research and classes were going, always mentioning how important he felt it is that we are bringing these practices to people with cancer and their caregivers.

His Holiness Lungtok Tenpai Nyima was the other elder who helped preserve the Bon tradition in exile in India. He was born in 1929 in the far eastern Tibetan province of Amdo. His Holiness was essential in my learning the yoga of *Instructions of the A.* Under his supervision, I did a 60-day retreat (a condensed version of the 100-day retreat by Shardza Rinpoche) at Menri Monastery in India, where he generously met with me daily, teaching and testing me. He did not allow me to electronically record any of my lessons, and the majority of the time, he wouldn't even allow me to bring my laptop, just the Tibetan text and pencil and paper. It was a wonderful experience and way to learn and train under his tutelage. In addition, Lopon Trinley Nyima met with me periodically to respond to some of the questions I still had, and, being younger than His Holiness, Lopon was able to show me himself how to perform the magical movements, which His Holiness would then test me on.

In addition to group practices and receiving teachings with His Holiness and Lopon once or twice a day, I would wake up every morning at 4 or 5 A.M. and practice four times a day on my own. My time at Menri—learning with these outstanding teachers, being around the monks, and having time to practice on my own, after which I could ask questions to make sure I was learning correctly—was an incredible opportunity that I still relish today. It has benefited me immensely in understanding these beautiful and profound yogic practices, and it is in that spirit that I bring them to you today.

Tibetan Yoga Comes to the West

Tenzin Wangyal Rinpoche was trained in the Bon tradition under Yongdzin Tenzin Namdak and His Holiness Lungtok Tenpai Nyima at Menri Monastery in India. He graduated as a geshe in 1986 and came to the West—Italy—in 1988 at the invitation of Namkhai Norbu Rinpoche. In 1991, he came to the United States through a Rice University Rockefeller Fellowship. In 1992, he founded Ligmincha Institute, with its main center in Virginia, to preserve the ancient Tibetan teachings, arts, and sciences, including the yogas, for future generations. Since coming to the West, Rinpoche has been emphasizing the importance of the five elements in his teachings. Among his many books, *Awakening the Sacred Body* presents the five *Tsa lung* yoga movements that relate to the five elements and the five breaths, making that work a good complement to the Tibetan yoga presented in this book.

Rinpoche has been my mentor and teacher since I met him in the Tibetan new year (*Losar*) of 1993. In 1994, I went to Virginia to begin my master's studies in Tibetan religions at the University of Virginia, after having learned the Tibetan yoga at Triten Norbutse the year before. When Rinpoche realized the extent of my interest in the Tibetan yogas, he generously offered to meet with me daily at 5 A.M. to discuss the Tibetan yoga teachings. He is the one who directed me to learn more from His Holiness at Menri monastery.

In 1994, Rinpoche began a seven-year training at Ligmincha Institute in Virginia that was composed of three-week retreats in the summer and included testing on the theory and practices. During these retreats, he would bring his teachers—either Yongdzin Tenzin Namdak or His Holiness Lungtok Tenpai Nyima—providing an amazing opportunity to learn from and spend time with them. This training was comprised of teachings from the causal vehicles, to the result vehicles of Sutra and Tantra, to Dzogchen, including the *Instructions of the A*. I was very happy to graduate in 2000, after being the main practice leader *(umdze)* had helped me to learn the practices deeply. Rinpoche also encouraged me to continue my academic training by pursuing a Ph.D. at Rice University. The seven-year Ligmincha training, together with my academic learning focusing on these practices and my trips to Triten Norbutse and Menri monastery mostly during the winter months, helped me continue to keep my practice and learning year-round. At the second summer retreat, Rinpoche asked me to start sharing the Tibetan yoga that I had learned in the monasteries with the retreat participants.

Ligmincha 16

In 2007, because of what I had learned in the monasteries, Tenzin Wangyal Rinpoche asked me to help condense the Tibetan Yoga of *Instructions of the A* together with two geshes, Tenzin Yangton and Tenzin Yeshe, during the summer retreat at Ligmincha Institute in Virginia. Although we had been teaching Tibetan yoga at the summer retreats since 2004, it was from *The Oral Transmission of Zhang Zhung*, which some people found difficult. Tenzin Wangyal Rinpoche felt the need to offer a Tibetan yoga set that was simple, yet complete and true to the tradition. That summer Rinpoche was teaching on the topic of developing inner heat, or *tummo*, using in particular a commentary by Shardza Rinpoche that mentioned the Tibetan Yoga of *Instructions of the A*. This provided the perfect opportunity to introduce this Tibetan yoga to our retreat participants, and Rinpoche was ready for the task. Over the three-week retreat, Rinpoche, the two geshes, and I condensed the 40 principal movements, following Rinpoche's guidance. We kept the one general, foundational movement, called *ngondro*, and then selected three movements for each of the five principles based on the five kinds of breath-energies and relating to the five elements and their five correlating chakras. And the result was what we have here in this book today, the Ligmincha 16.

Being a part of this process was both fascinating and an honor, as well as a wonderful way to deepen my own practice. We taught the Ligmincha 16 to the whole group of about 80 at the retreat in our first test run. The practice was very well received as a complete set of Tibetan yoga that was also "doable." Since then, we have taught the Ligmincha 16 at other Ligmincha summer retreats and in Tibetan yoga retreats and trainings in the United States, Latin America, and Europe.

Thanks to this wonderful lineage of teachers, and the kindness of His Holiness Lungtok Tenpai Nyima, Yongdzin Tenzin Namdak, and Tenzin Wangyal Rinpoche, these teachings are now here for you to practice and benefit from in your everyday life.

CHAPTER 4

The Modern Yogi

In the Bon tradition, yogis practiced different kinds of meditation and breathings for years before learning the yogic movements. This is why ancient texts, curricula, and meditation manuals first start with calming and focusing one's mind, training the breath, and learning the subtle body. Then they incorporate the yoga movements, which is the methodology I have utilized in this book.

As I was learning this Tibetan yoga at Menri Monastery, Lopon Trinley Nyima described how the movements were designed by yogis who realized that incorporating such body practices enhanced their already-trained focus and also helped them release obstacles that had prevented them from remaining in their natural, or *A*, state of mind. They also used them to strengthen and rebalance their health when they were ill. These yogis would sometimes practice in isolation in a cave or in a monastery. They centered their day and life around their spiritual practice, including these yogas.

But what about the normal, everyday person who needs to find time to squeeze some of these practices into their daily routine? Sometimes we don't have the time we want to dedicate to our formal practice because we overslept, had to work late, needed to take our children to school or afterschool activities, or any number of perfectly normal and unavoidable reasons. To help make Tibetan yoga a realistic part of your daily routine, I will provide a few models of practice that vary according to the amount of time you have available. As for the time of the day to practice, it depends on when you can make the time. Some people prefer early morning before they start their daily activities. I think that is a good time as long as you are not in a hurry to finish and get on with your day but instead feel that you are "charging your batteries" for the day. The end of the day can also be good, but do not wait until you are very tired, otherwise your meditation will not be clear, with a feeling of dullness or a "cloudy mind." I know many people who prefer to practice at noon or take a break from work in mid-morning or afternoon. All are good times for the modern yogi.

In general, I recommend choosing one principal movement from each of the five sets for each breath. Then you can have a simple practice of five total movements (or six, if we count the foundational movement, or *ngondro*). Or you can choose the movements you feel you most need at that time. But no matter what movements you choose or the amount of time you are able to practice, it is important to center and connect with yourself every day.

It is also important to always start with your intention for the practice and to conclude it with the dedication or sharing the benefits of your practice, "pouring nectar into the ocean," so that everyone can benefit, including yourself.

The intention and the sharing of benefits make up the outer frame of a practice session, and there are several options for the inner content of the practice. Beyond the time that you have available, you can also choose to focus on a primarily seated meditative practice or one that includes the yoga movements—some practitioners even include standing and jumping. I will give you options for both.

If you have just 5 to 7 minutes to practice:

1. Take about a minute to settle into your posture and set your intention.

2. Perform the Nine Breathings of Purification (p. 16).

3. Rest in the meditative, or *A*, state of mind for about a minute or two.

4. Share the benefits of your practice, which could take less than a minute.

OR

1. Take about a minute to settle into your posture and set your intention.

2. Perform the Nine Breathings of Purification (p. 16).

3. Perform the Foundational Movement (p. 26).

4. Rest in the meditative, or *A*, state of mind for about a minute.

5. Share the benefits of your practice.

If you have around 15 minutes to practice:

1. Take a minute or two to settle into your posture and set your intention.

2. Perform the Nine Breathings of Purification (p. 16).

3. Perform the Connecting with your Heart meditation (p. 5).

4. Share the benefits of your practice.

OR

1. Take a minute or two to settle into your posture and set your intention.

2. Bring your attention to your breath and start the simple conscious breathing (p. 5) and then perform the Nine Breathings of Purification (p. 16).

3. Perform the Foundational Movement (p. 26).

4. Perform one movement of your choosing from each of the five sets, for a total of five movements.

5. Rest, sitting or lying down (*shavasana*), in a meditative, or *A*, state of mind for a minute or two.

6. Sit upright, assume the five-point posture, and conclude by sharing the benefits of your practice.

If you have 30 minutes to practice:

1. Take a minute or two to settle into your posture and set your intention.

2. Perform the Nine Breathings of Purification (p. 16).

3. Perform the Connecting with Your Heart meditation (p. 5).

4. Perform the three Principal Movements that purify your upper torso and more closely connect you to your heart center.

5. Rest, sitting cross-legged or in the five-point posture, in a meditative, or *A*, state of mind for about two minutes.

6. Share the benefits of your practice.

OR

1. Take a minute or two to settle into your posture and set your intention.

2. Bring your attention to your breath, start the simple conscious breathing (p. 5), and then perform the Nine Breathings of Purification (p. 16).

3. Start the Experiential Run through Your Chakras (p. 20).

4. Perform the Foundational Movement (p. 26).

5. Perform one movement of your choosing from each of the five sets, for a total of five movements.

6. Rest, sitting or lying down, in a meditative, or *A*, state of mind for about two minutes.

7. Sit upright, assume the five-point posture, and conclude by sharing the benefit of your practice.

OR here's a third option, if you want to include all the magical movements in a short practice.

1. Take a minute or two to settle into your posture and set your intention.

2. Bring your attention to your breath and start the simple conscious breathing (p. 5) and then perform the Nine Breathings of Purification (p. 16).

3. Perform the Foundational Movement (p. 26).

4. Perform the 15 Principal Movements (p. 29).

5. Rest, sitting or lying down, in a meditative, or *A*, state of mind for about two minutes.

6. Sit upright in the cross-legged position or the five-point posture and conclude by sharing the benefits of your practice.

If you have 45–60 minutes, you could do a full practice.

1. Take a minute or two to settle into your posture and set your intention.

2. Bring your attention to your breath and start the simple conscious breathing (p. 5) and then perform the Nine Breathings of Purification (p. 16).

3. Perform the Connecting with Your Heart meditation (p. 5).

4. Start your Experiential Run through Your Chakras (p. 20).

5. Perform the Foundational Movement (p. 26).

6. Perform the 15 Principal Movements (p. 29).

7. Rest, sitting or lying down, in a meditative, or *A*, state of mind.

8. Sit upright in the cross-legged position or the five-point posture and take a moment to notice how you feel in each of your chakras and the whole central channel.

9. Conclude by sharing the benefits of your practice.

These are just a few suggestions for bringing a formal time for practice into your life. As it becomes part of your healthy daily routine, you will be able to integrate that *A* state of mind into your whole day.

And even on those days when you feel you don't have five minutes to practice, take a moment as you wake up to set your intention for the day and do some simple conscious breathing—inhaling and exhaling a couple of times—reconnecting yourself to your heart or inner home and readying yourself to start your day.

It is important to keep some sense of awareness throughout the day, which we sometimes call *informal practice*. Bring awareness to your daily activities with meditation moments, or "meditation pills," by consciously focusing on your breath for a few moments several times during the day.

It may be helpful to use the STOP formula, which I first heard about from Susan Bauer-Wu, who is now the president of Mind & Life Institute:

Stop.

Take a few deep, conscious breaths.

Open your heart and observe how you feel.

Proceed—or, if you are not ready to proceed, continue observing and breathing consciously for a time.

Throughout the day, you can use STOP in different situations.

- Whenever you wash your hands, use the time to wash your mind as well. As you focus on lathering and rinsing, take slow breaths and imagine that you are also cleansing your mind.

- While sitting, stretch your arms upward. As you lengthen your back, breathe deeply through your nose, into your belly, and back out through your nose. Lower your arms, place them on your lap, and take a few deep, calm breaths.

- When you pull up to a stoplight in the car, do as the Vietnamese master Thich Nhat Hanh says and thank the red light, and then take the opportunity to connect to yourself: Ignore your phone, turn off the radio, and pause to breathe in peace and release anxious thoughts. Of course, you need to do this one with your eyes open.

Acknowledging how hectic our lives are and having tools to assist us in our formal and informal practice is what makes us modern yogis. In one of our recent Tibetan yoga studies, we found that you needed to do formal practice more than twice—at least three times a week—to keep the benefits.[1] And, of course, try to keep up with your daily informal practice with the meditation moments, or "meditation pills," or STOP formula.

You can take these meditation pills as if they were aspirin, when your head hurts or when you feel stress, or, even better, as an antibiotic, four times a day, without needing to wait for that stress to be imminent.

So, just as you engage formally and informally in your practice during the day, at night, or right before you go to sleep, also take a moment to do a few conscious breaths and use them to wash your mind. Then, bring your attention to your heart center and, with an inner smile, fall asleep. In this way, you can keep your practice during the cycle of day and night.

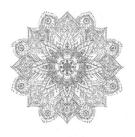

Afterword

Sharing from the Heart

Tibetan practitioners conclude their Tibetan yoga sessions with a dedication prayer or sharing the benefits of one's practice, as I mentioned in step 5. With the dedication, you actualize the intention of relieving the suffering of others by sharing the benefits of the practice with all sentient beings.

I have always found this part of the practice very powerful, even when a prayer is not recited with it. As I describe at the end of Chapter 2 and in the models of practice in Chapter 4, it is important to share the benefits of your practice at the end of a session. And, as Yongdzin Tenzin Namdak has taught, you can also do this during the day, with informal sessions, and at the end of the day. With that in mind, I would like to share a prayer I composed in

English for my children, which we recite together every night. You might find it helpful too.

I pray that all my actions of body, speech, and mind

Be for the benefit of all sentient beings.

May all my actions be good and none of my actions be bad.

May all beings be happy, may all beings be happy, and may all beings be happy.

My kids suggested that as we recite "may all beings be happy" three times, we gradually extend our arms more for each repetition, and in the last one give each other a big, warmhearted hug. Then we say *good night*!

My hope is that these Tibetan yogas, in both formal and informal practice, will help you heal externally and internally as much as they warm your heart toward others and yourself.

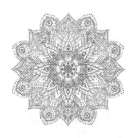

Resources

Support Materials and References

Connecting with Your Heart—An introductory meditation using mind and breath to connect more deeply to yourself. Covers mind, breath, and visualization.

https://www.mdanderson.org/patients-family/diagnosis-treatment/care-centers-clinics/integrative-medicine-center/audio_and_video.html

The long version is entitled "Power of Breath I," and the short version is entitled "Tibetan Meditation: Connect with Your Heart."

Clearing Inner Obstacles: 9 Breathings of Purification

https://www.mdanderson.org/patients-family/diagnosis-treatment/care-centers-clinics/integrative-medicine-center/audio_and_video.html

Ligmincha Atri Trul Khor
  Video by Vision is Mind Productions
  https://youtu.be/goz6tRLhbEg

Note: there may be some slight differences in the way the movements are performed in the video. The most updated version is the one in the book.

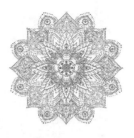

Endnotes

Preface

1. M. Alejandro Chaoul, "Magical Movements (*'phrul 'khor*): Ancient Yogic Practices in the Bon Religion and Contemporary Medical Perspectives," Ph.D. dissertation, Rice University, Houston, TX, May 2006.

Introduction

1. Chaoul, "Magical Movements," pp. 16–17. I want to particularly thank Yongdzin Tenzin Namdak and Lopon Trinely Nyima for the numerous discussions about the significance of the Tibetan meaning of *trul* and *khor* in the context of these *trul khor* yogic practices.

2. Chaoul, "Magical Movements," p. 17. I want to thank Khenpo Tenpa Yungdrung for our conversations and his clarification on *trul* as magic in this context.

3. Michael Murphy, *The Future of the Body*, New York, N.Y.: Penguin Books, 1992.

4. These studies were conducted at MD Anderson's Integrative Medicine Program, where the aim, following Engel's seminal paper in *Science* in 1977, is to provide healing focused not just on the physical (i.e., biomedicine), but also on the psychosocial-spiritual aspects of the person, which sometimes seem to be forgotten in conventional allopathic medicine (Engel 1977, where he proposes the need for a bio-psycho-social-spiritual model to supplement the current biomedical model). George L. Engel, "The Need for a New Medical Model: A Challenge for Biomedicine," *Science*, 1977 Apr 8;196(4286):129–36.

5. Lorenzo Cohen, et al., "Psychological adjustment and sleep quality in a randomized trial of the effects of a Tibetan yoga intervention in patients with lymphoma," *Cancer*, 2004 May 15;100(10):2253–60, https://doi.org/10.1002/cncr.20236.

6. Alejandro Chaoul, et al., "Mind-body practices in cancer care," *Current Oncology Reports*, 2014 Dec, 16(12):417, https://doi.org/10.1007/s11912-014-0417-x.

7. Kathrin Milbury, et al., "Couple-based Tibetan yoga program for lung cancer patients and their caregivers," *Psycho-Oncology*, 2015 Jan;24(1):117–20, https://doi.org/10.1002/pon.3588.

8. Alejandro Chaoul, et al., "An Exploration of the Effects of Tibetan Yoga on Patient's Quality of Life and Experience of Lymphoma: An Experimental Embedded Mixed Methods Study," *Journal of Alternative and Complementary Medicine*, 2014 May 7, 20(5):A133.

9. Suzanne C. Danhauer, et al., "Evidence Supports Incorporating Yoga Alongside Conventional Cancer Treatment

for Women with Breast Cancer," *Breast Diseases*, 2015 Jan 1, 26(3):189–193, https://doi.org/10.1016/j.breast-dis.2015.07.036.

10. Isabel Leal, et al., "An Exploration of the Effects of Tibetan Yoga on Patients' Psychological Well-Being and Experience of Lymphoma: An Experimental Embedded Mixed Methods Study," *Journal of Mixed Methods Research*, 2016 May 2, 12(1):31–54, https://doi.org/10.1177/1558689816645005.

11. Alejandro Chaoul et al., "Randomized trial of Tibetan yoga in patients with breast cancer undergoing chemotherapy." *Cancer*, 2018 Jan 1, 124(1):36–45, https://doi.org/10.1002/cncr.30938.

12. In this setting, "mind-body" refers to the experience of our existence as a whole and to not having our mind isolated from our body. The Tibetan traditions also explain what I like to call the missing link between "mind" and "body"—"energy" (*rtsal*), which is mostly expressed as speech and breath. In the Western clinical research setting, an intervention refers to a particular program's design (in this case, Tibetan yoga) for use with a particular population (in this case, cancer patients) to help improve an aspect of their health.

13. Bruce Lawrence, "Transformation," *Critical Terms for Religious Studies*, ed. Mark Taylor, Chicago and London: University of Chicago Press, 1998, p. 335.

Chapter 1

1. Herbert Benson and Miriam Z. Klipper, *The Relaxation Response*, New York: HarperCollins, 2000.

2. This is a simplified version of the Internal *Tsa lung of the Mother Tantra*, inspired in the oral teachings of

Tenzin Wangyal Rinpoche. For the internal *Tsa lung* see Rinpoche's *Awakening the Sacred Body*, New York and Carlsbad, CA: Hay House, 2011, pp. 78–80.

Chapter 2

1. The text we used was Shardza Tashi Gyaltsen (*rShar rdza bkhra shis rgyal mtshan*), "The Enhancing Magical Movements of the Play of the Illusory Body" (*Bogs 'don 'phrul 'khor sgyu ma'i rol mo*), from *The Complete Perfection's Self-Arising of the three Enlightened Bodies*, (*rDzogs pa Chen po Sku gsum rang shar*), ed. Khedup Gyatso, Delhi: Tibetan Bonpo Monastic Centre, 1974.

Chapter 3

1. Bru-sgom rGyal-ba gyung-drung, *The Stages of A-Khrid Meditation: Dzogchen Practice of the Bon Tradition*, trans. Per Kvaerne and Thubten Rikey, New Delhi: Paljor, 2002. The A-Khrid teachings regarding the Ultimate Origin-(A) is believed to have a historical source in the great lama rMe'u dGongs-mdzod (1038–1096). This translation presents a condensed version of his original composition, written by Bru-sgom rGyal-ba gyung-drung (1242–1296).

Chapter 4

1. Chaoul et al., "Randomized trial of Tibetan yoga." (short title) *Cancer*, 2018 Jan 1, 124(1):36–45, https://doi.org/10.1002/cncr.30938.

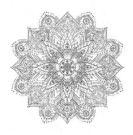

Acknowledgments

I am very grateful for the causes and conditions that have aligned to help me write this book, and for all the wonderful people who contributed along the way. I am especially grateful to the teachers and protectors of these teachings, without whom these practices and this book would not have been possible.

It was through Namkhai Norbu Rinpoche that I first heard that Tibetan Yoga existed. He called it *Yantra Yoga* and taught from the *Union of Sun and Moon* text. I was able to learn those practices from him and Fabio Andrico. I thank them for opening this magical door.

Triten Norbutse Monastery in Nepal has been a very sacred place for me, and it was there that I first learned the Tibetan Yoga from the Bon tradition. My gratitude to Yongdzin Tenzin Namdak, Khenpo Nyima Wangyal, and Khenpo Tenpa Yungdrung. And to Yungdrung Tenzin, then a young monk who had recently arrived from Amdo, who taught me those first Bon magical movements.

I cannot find enough words to thank Tenzin Wangyal Rinpoche, my continuous spiritual and academic mentor. He noticed how I fell in love with these magical movements and guided me to deepen my study and practice, not only with him but also with his teachers in the United States and in their monasteries.

Rinpoche also wrote the foreword for this book and kindly drew, at my request, the calligraphy of the homage of the *A-tri Trul khor* text and the calligraphy of the *A*.

His Holiness Lungtok Tenpai Nyima, and Lopon Trinley Nyima, from Menri Monastery in India deserve most of the credit for teaching me the Tibetan Yoga from the *Instructions of the A*. I cherish and thank them from the very depth of my heart for their commitment to teaching and guiding me during the couple of months I spent at the monastery and on my many subsequent visits with each one in the United States and at the monastery.

Geshe Tenzin Yangton, Geshe Tenzin Yeshe, and I teamed up under the direction of Tenzin Wangyal Rinpoche to condense those magical movements of the *Instructions of the A* into the Ligmincha 16 that you see in this book. I am honored to have practiced and learned from them, and to have co-taught so many times at Ligmincha International.

My immense gratitude goes to Patty Gift from Hay House, whom I met—perhaps serendipitously—on a bus ride to Omega Institute over a decade ago. Since then she has been the main sounding board and fairy godmother of this book.

Lisa Cheng has been my main editor from Hay House, helping me over the last year and a half with countless back-and-forth e-mails to bring this book to its present form. An enormous thanks to her and all the Hay House team, from copy editors to marketing, including Nancy Elgin, KB Mello, Marlene Robinson, Anne Barthel, Blaine Todfield, and others behind the scenes.

As a former art director in an advertising agency, I know the importance of graphics in any book. I am very grateful to Howie Severson for designing the beautiful cover and Bryn Starr Best for the elegant interior design.

The amazing multiple-exposure photos of the magical movements are the artwork of Andreas Zihler from Zurich. Thank you so much for your time, expertise, and kind disposition to have these photos illustrate this book.

Tom Maroshegyi has been a good friend and student, who created and manages my website. I greatly appreciate the many photos of still poses and hand details that he took for this book when I was teaching in Esalen. Big thanks!

Angel Alcalá very kindly gave me permission to use the beautiful photo of His Holiness Lungtok Tenpai Nyima for the dedication of this book. *¡Muchas Gracias!*

My *thug je che* to Lhari-la Kalsang Nyima, who was happy to let me use his illustrations of the channels and chakras.

Volker Graf, also a friend and student who is very dedicated to *Trul khor,* trained with me in Europe and filmed the magical movements in Gran Canaria. He did a wonderful job editing the film, and the link is provided for you in the Resources at the end of the book. *Vielen Dank* to you and Vision is Mind Prod.

I want to thank Mark Adamcik from UT TV who has recorded my numerous MD Anderson meditation audios and videos. You can find them at the MD Anderson Integrative Medicine website, also provided in the Resources section of this book.

Friends and students read versions or parts of the book and contributed to this more polished version. I want to extend my gratitude to Rob Patzig, Anne Forbes, Laura Shekerjian, and Amy Hertz. Other friends, teachers, and colleagues whom I admire read it and wrote endorsements for this book: Roshi Joan Halifax, Sharon Salzberg, Elissa Epel, Lorenzo Cohen, Susan Bauer-Wu, Jeff

Kripal, Cyndi Lee, Mary Taylor, and Richard Freeman. A deep bow and my profound gratitude to each one of you.

A heartfelt *gracias* to my family, Erika, Matías Namdak *y* Karina Dawa, who are such an important part of my life and have accompanied me in many of my dharma-related trips and have met many of my teachers. Our evenings usually end with reciting the prayer included in the afterword of this book.

To my mom, Susi Reich, who early in my life opened my eyes and mind to different perspectives, and to the role of what today we call integrative medicine. Thanks for all your inroads into new fields, even if they seemed "weird" at that time.

I also thank my dad, Fred Chaoul, through whom I entered the world of people with cancer and got a better understanding of the human aspect of it. Both he and his wife, Mirtha, have been very supportive of my work.

Last but not least, I want to thank my in-laws, Katy Chamberlain and Delfino De la Garza. Katy has been a strong foundation for the whole family, and I always feel her comforting support toward my work and elected path of life. Delfino, one of my most enthusiastic cheerleaders who passed away a few years ago, came to some of my Tibetan yoga retreats in Mexico and even early morning meditations in the cold of La Guasteca, Monterrey. I can visualize you in the sky, like the last time I visited you: sitting in a hospital bed, opening your arms to greet me with the kind heart and big smile that characterized you. This book is also for you.

Thank you, *thugjeche, vielen Dank,* and *mil gracias* to all of you!!!

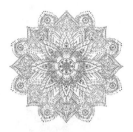

About the Author

D R. ALEJANDRO CHAOUL is an Assistant Professor and the Director of Education at the Integrative Medicine Program at the University of Texas MD Anderson Cancer Center, where he conducts Tibetan meditation and movement classes, clinic, and research to assess the effects of Tibetan yoga practices and mind-body techniques in people with cancer and their caregivers. He is also a Senior Teacher at The 3 Doors, an international organization founded by Tenzin Wangyal Rinpoche with the goal of transforming lives through meditation. Dr. Chaoul has studied in the Tibetan tradition for over 25 years with His Holiness Lungtok Tenpai Nyima, Yongdzin Tenzin Namdak, and Tenzin Wangyal Rinpoche. He has completed the seven-year training at Ligmincha Institute and holds a Ph.D. in Tibetan Religions from Rice University. Dr. Chaoul is director for research of Ligmincha International, and teaches meditation and Tibetan Yoga workshops nationally, as well as internationally in Latin America and Europe. He is the founding director of the Mind, Body, Spirit Institute at The Jung Center of Houston and has been recognized as a Fellow of the Mind & Life Institute.

He is the author of *Chöd Practice in the Bon Tradition*, and you can visit him online at **alechaoul.com**.

Hay House Titles of Related Interest

YOU CAN HEAL YOUR LIFE, the movie,
starring Louise Hay & Friends
(available as an online streaming video)
www.hayhouse.com/louise-movie

THE SHIFT, the movie,
starring Dr. Wayne W. Dyer
(available as an online streaming video)
www.hayhouse.com/the-shift-movie

***

*AWAKENING THE LUMINOUS MIND: Tibetan Meditation for Inner Peace
and Joy,* by Tenzin Wangyal Rinpoche

AWAKENING THE SACRED BODY: Tibetan Yogas of Breath and Movement,
by Tenzin Wangyal Rinpoche

*SECRETS OF MEDITATION: A Practical Guide to Inner Peace and Personal
Transformation,* by davidji

*YOU HAVE 4 MINUTES TO CHANGE YOUR LIFE: Simple 4-Minute
Meditations for Inspiration, Transformation, and True Bliss,*
by Rebekah Borucki

All of the above are available at your local bookstore,
or may be ordered by contacting Hay House (see next page).

***

We hope you enjoyed this Hay House book. If you'd like to receive our online catalog featuring additional information on Hay House books and products, or if you'd like to find out more about the Hay Foundation, please contact:

Hay House, Inc., P.O. Box 5100, Carlsbad, CA 92018-5100
(760) 431-7695 or (800) 654-5126
(760) 431-6948 (fax) or (800) 650-5115 (fax)
www.hayhouse.com® • www.hayfoundation.org

———

Published in Australia by: Hay House Australia Pty. Ltd.,
18/36 Ralph St., Alexandria NSW 2015
Phone: 612-9669-4299 • *Fax:* 612-9669-4144
www.hayhouse.com.au

Published in the United Kingdom by: Hay House UK, Ltd.,
The Sixth Floor, Watson House, 54 Baker Street, London W1U 7BU
Phone: +44 (0)20 3927 7290 • *Fax:* +44 (0)20 3927 7291
www.hayhouse.co.uk

Published in India by: Hay House Publishers India,
Muskaan Complex, Plot No. 3, B-2, Vasant Kunj, New Delhi 110 070
Phone: 91-11-4176-1620 • *Fax:* 91-11-4176-1630
www.hayhouse.co.in

———

Access New Knowledge.
Anytime. Anywhere.

Learn and evolve at your own pace
with the world's leading experts.

www.hayhouseU.com